BASIC OPHTHALMOSCOPY

OPHTHALMOSCOPIC DIAGNOSIS
IN SYSTEMIC DISORDERS

Also by Mr. Rosen:

FLUORESCENCE PHOTOGRAPHY OF THE EYE

A Manual of Dynamic Clinical Ocular Fundus Pathology

Basic
Ophthalmoscopy

Ophthalmoscopic Diagnosis
in Systemic Disorders

EMANUEL S. ROSEN

M.D., B.Sc., F.R.C.S.(Ed.), F.R.P.S.

*Senior Ophthalmic Registrar, Manchester Royal
Eye Hospital, Manchester, England*

and

HANNAH SAVIR, M.D.

*Senior Ophthalmic Surgeon, Beilinson Hospital,
University of Tel Aviv, Israel*

London : Butterworths

ENGLAND: BUTTERWORTH & CO. (PUBLISHERS) LTD.
LONDON: 88 Kingsway, WC2B 6AB

AUSTRALIA: BUTTERWORTH & CO. (AUSTRALIA) LTD.
SYDNEY: 586 Pacific Highway, NSW 2067
MELBOURNE: 343 Little Collins Street, 3000
BRISBANE: 240 Queen Street, 4000

CANADA: BUTTERWORTH & CO. (CANADA) LTD.
TORONTO: 14 Curity Avenue, 374

NEW ZEALAND: BUTTERWORTH & CO. (NEW ZEALAND) LTD.
WELLINGTON: 26-28 Waring Taylor Street, 1
AUCKLAND: 35 High Street, 1

SOUTH AFRICA: BUTTERWORTH & CO. (SOUTH AFRICA) (PTY) LTD.
DURBAN: 152-154 Gale Street

Suggested U.D.C. No. 617.7-072.1

ISBN 0 407 11370 3

Made and printed in Great Britain by
William Clowes & Sons, Limited
London, Beccles and Colchester

Contents

Preface

The purpose of this book is to provide the physician, medical student and student of ophthalmic optics with a basic guide to the art and science of ophthalmoscopy. Advantage is taken of a major development in ophthalmology in the past decade, fluorescein angiography, to correlate ophthalmoscopic findings recorded by colour photography with the detailed findings revealed and recorded by fundus angiography. The microscopic detail of angiograms and the dynamic information gained about fundus physiology and pathology, together provide a more active appreciation of the ophthalmoscopic view.

An introduction to ophthalmoscopy and ophthalmoscopes is followed by an ophthalmoscopic consideration of normal fundus anatomy. The pathologic fundus is discussed in general terms with an emphasis on the reasons why lesions appear as they do. A classification of fundus disorders embraces this section and is based on the limited ways the fundus can respond to a wide variety of disorders. For the uninitiated, a simple guide to interpretation of fluorescein angiograms completes the introduction.

Limitations on space and the desirability of pairing each colour illustration with a single meaningful angiogram wherever possible, governed the selection of material for the section on specific disorders. Natural incidence of disease in the community has prompted wider coverage of the retinopathies of diabetes, hypertension and optic nerve disorders from other less frequently encountered items. It was not our intention to present an ophthalmoscopic view of every known retinopathy, this being the province of a comprehensive and expensive reference textbook. Rather has it been our intention to illustrate some *principles* of ophthalmoscopic diagnosis as seen in several different types of disorder and most often when the fundus signs were an expression of systemic disease.

The restricted area of the fundus that it is possible to cover with a single photograph is a limitation that is not our wish to disguise, but rather to utilize by concentration on a particular feature, thus emphasizing principles which will guide readers to a more satisfying and productive use of their ophthalmoscopes.

Manchester   E. S. ROSEN

Colour transparencies

Limitations imposed by letterpress reproduction of coloured illustrations must inevitably result in some loss of detail. Examination through a magnifier will show that the images are composed of integrated patterns of very fine coloured dots.

For those who wish to see the fundus as the ophthalmologist sees it through his ophthalmoscope, the publishers have made arrangements with The Slide Centre Limited to produce economically priced sets of colour transparencies duplicated from the photographs made in the fundus camera. These duplicates carry transparent dye images of a virtually grainless pattern and, viewed by transmitted light, present views of the fundus almost exactly as would be seen through an ophthalmoscope.

The transparencies are supplied in standard card mounts suitable for use in any of the many commercially obtainable viewers or 35 mm still projectors, thus catering for those who wish to study privately and for the tutor who is enabled to project the views to a class.

The sets of 48 mounted slides are obtainable direct from

The Slide Centre Limited,
Portman House,
Brodrick Street,
London S.W.17

Please note that Butterworths do not supply the slides.

SECTION I

Ophthalmoscopy, Ophthalmoscopic Anatomy, Ophthalmoscopic Pathology and Fluorescein Angiography

1—Ophthalmoscopy

Ophthalmoscopy, a method of clinical examination of the fundus of the eye, is a most important diagnostic technique. Acquisition of expertise in fundus examination by ophthalmoscopy requires diligent practice and careful instruction. An appreciation of normal fundus anatomy and its variations is a necessary beginning upon which a student can build a personal knowledge of fundus pathology, capable of yielding invaluable diagnostic information.

The fundus of the eye affords a privileged situation where the peripheral circulation may be viewed in the living state. In the past 120 years this opportunity has been used by physiologists, physicians and ophthalmologists to study normal and abnormal processes with both local and systemic significance.

It was in 1851 that von Helmholtz invented the ophthalmoscope. The invention arose from an attempt by him to demonstrate to his class the nature of the glow of the reflected light sometimes seen in the eyes of animals such as the cat. When the great ophthalmologist von Graefe first saw the fundus of the living eye, with its optic disc and blood vessels, his face flushed with excitement and he cried 'Helmholtz has unfolded to us a new world'.

The ophthalmoscope of von Helmholtz used an external light source and a mirror with a central aperture through which the observer looked from the non-reflecting side of the mirror. In 1885 Dennett introduced the self-illuminated electric ophthalmoscope. Because light which leaves an eye is necessarily reflected in the direction from which it came, the pupil appears black. If, however, an observer's eye is placed to intercept these reflected rays then the interior of the observed eye will appear illuminated, provided that there is a sufficiently good light source for observation. Placing the observer's eye in the path of the returning rays through a perforation in the mirror, which is used to reflect the light into the eye under observation, allows the interior of the eye to be examined. This is the basic theory of ophthalmoscopy.

A year after von Helmholtz's invention in 1851 of the direct ophthalmoscope Ruete developed the indirect method of ophthalmoscopy.

DIRECT OPHTHALMOSCOPY

Direct ophthalmoscopic image

Nature. The image is virtual and erect (*Diagram 1*).

Magnification is about × 15 if the observed eye is emmetropic. If the observed eye is short-sighted or myopic, the magnification is greater,

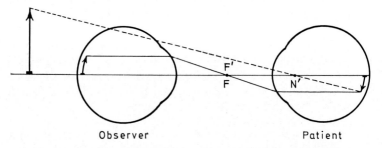

Observer   Patient

Diagram 1. Optical principles of the direct method of ophthalmoscopy

depending on the degree of myopia. In hypermetropia or long-sightedness the image is correspondingly smaller or less magnified.

Field of view subtends approximately 10 degrees in diameter (instrument variation).

Fundus area capable of visualization is 60 to 70 per cent of the total fundus area of an emmetropic eye, less than this in a myopic eye and rather more in a hypermetropic eye. The remaining fundus can be seen by the method of indirect ophthalmoscopy, if the sophisticated technique of scleral indentation is employed (this is of special interest to ophthalmologists).

Medial opacities provide an awkward obstruction to the view of the fundus.

Image brightness depends on the source of illumination. Battery-powered direct ophthalmoscopes provide a satisfactory but generally low level of illumination. Mains-powered electric ophthalmoscopes on the other hand allow the intensity of illumination to be varied from dim to very bright levels by the use of a rheostat. The transparency of the media of the eye also influence image brightness.

Monochrome ophthalmoscopy. Coloured filters are easily incorporated to offer, for example, a red-free view of the fundus.

Stereoscopy. Stereoscopic images are not possible with a conventional direct ophthalmoscope which is monocular.

Working distance of the direct ophthalmoscope is 1 to 5 centimetres from the observed eye.

Portability varies from the highly portable pen-like pocket ophthalmoscopes now available, to the less mobile mains-operated ophthalmoscopes. There is no doubt that the fountain pen-like, highly portable, pocket ophthalmoscope offers greatest convenience to the physician.

Availability. The complexity of direct ophthalmoscopes available on the commercial markets corresponds to their price. For practical purposes and general use the simpler instruments are more satisfactory. Dioptric corrections in the ophthalmoscope should be available from +20 through to −20. Beyond these limits alternative methods of fundus examination are indicated. In extreme ametropia the subject's own glasses should be worn to provide automatic correction of the refractive error.

INDIRECT OPHTHALMOSCOPY

Indirect (binocular) ophthalmoscopic image

Nature. The image is inverted and real. The technique is called indirect because the fundus is observed through a condensing lens (*Diagram 2*). The distance from the observer to the image formed by the condensing lens will depend on the observer's own refractive error.

Magnification. In contrast to direct ophthalmoscopy it is very little affected by the patient's refractive error but is determined by the power of the condensing lens. A commonly used 20-diopter lens affords $\times 3\frac{1}{2}$ magnification.

Field of View. With the 20-diopter lens, approximately 37 degree diameter field (that is, the field of view is at least 13 times greater than the field of view offered by the direct ophthalmoscope).

$$\frac{\text{Area of direct ophthalmoscope field}}{\text{Area of indirect ophthalmoscope field}} \propto \frac{\text{radius of d.o.f.}^2}{\text{radius of i.o.f.}^2} = \frac{5^2}{18^2} = \frac{1}{13}$$

Fundus area capable of visualization is 70–80 per cent but the technique of scleral indentation will bring the whole of the fundus into view.

5

Medial opacities are penetrated surprisingly well by this method.

Stereoscopy. Unless the patient's pupil is very small, a stereoscopic view is obtained.

Image brightness depends on the light source, which is usually mains operated through a transformer and rheostat and therefore can be varied to the observer's satisfaction.

Instruments available. Indirect ophthalmoscopy can be performed either monocularly or binocularly. The binocular instrument whose

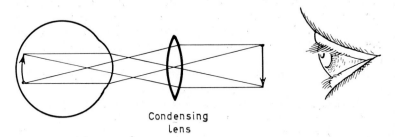

Condensing
Lens

Diagram 2. Optics of indirect ophthalmoscopy

features have been described above, offers the advantage of a stereoscopic image. The instrument is either worn on a headband or mounted on a spectacle frame. Thus the observer's hands are free but for the necessity of holding the condensing lens. A monocular indirect ophthalmoscope is usually hand-held, leaving no free hand for indentation.

An ophthalmologist may find many indications for the use of an indirect ophthalmoscope. In particular, he may use it to advantage to view the fundus through cloudy refractive media, in ametropia, in children and in retinal detachment work. On the other hand, the physician has little recourse to use this instrument, despite its advantages in the above-mentioned circumstances. The modern self-illuminated direct ophthalmoscope is the instrument of choice for the general medical student and the physician.

CLINICAL TECHNIQUE OF DIRECT OPHTHALMOSCOPY

The pupil

Dilatation of the pupil facilitates satisfactory ophthalmoscopy. The less experienced the observer, the greater the truth in this statement. Pupillary dilatation for diagnostic purposes should be undertaken with a short-acting mydriatic such as cyclopentolate (Mydrilate). At the conclusion of the fundus examination the pupil should be constricted by instillation of pilocarpine 2 per cent drops. In an iris which is heavily pigmented (brown) it is usually much more difficult to dilate the pupil than in one which is lightly pigmented (blue). There should be little hesitation in dilating pupils for the purpose of

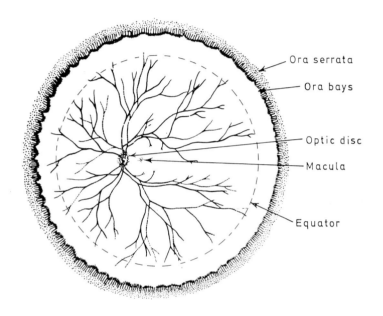

Diagram 3. Topographic view of fundus

ophthalmoscopy, but some precautions should be borne in mind because of the very occasional danger of an attack of acute closed-angle glaucoma. Clinical indications that this untoward event may be a possibility, include (1) age—it occurs in patients generally over 40 but usually over 50 years of age; (2) anterior chamber depth—it occurs in an eye which possesses a shallow anterior chamber. Gauging the depth of an anterior chamber, that is the distance between cornea and iris, is a matter of practice by observation; (3) a history of the patient having suffered intermittent attacks of blurred vision associated with haloes and aching sensations in the eye. In all cases of doubt about the effects of pupillary dilation, an experienced opinion should be sought.

7

Preliminary observations

With a +5 to +10-diopter lens, in the direct ophthalmoscope viewing aperture, the observer should examine the patient's eye from a distance of some 10 to 20 centimetres. By this means, opacities in the refractive media of the eye will appear as contrasting black against the red glow of the fundus (red reflex). Thus corneal, lenticular and vitreous opacities will be noted and will reduce confusion which otherwise would arise from the difficulties they cause in viewing the fundus. It should also be remembered that such opacities, particularly in the vitreous, may be the product of fundus changes and therefore may be of diagnostic significance (for example vitreous haemorrhage in diabetic retinopathy).

Fundus examination

A systematic approach to fundus examination is to be recommended. The optic disc is the natural starting point before moving temporally to examine the macula. By following the course of the principal radiating branches of the central retinal artery emerging from the optic disc, the quadrants of the posterior fundus can be covered and subsequently the peripheral fundus can be studied (*Diagram 3*).

2—Ophthalmoscopic Anatomy

NORMAL FUNDUS

A topographic view of a normal fundus, as seen with the ophthalmo-scope, is depicted in *Diagram 3 and Figure 1* (Section III). The optic nerve head with its radiating blood vessels is the key feature. Placed to the nasal side of the mid line the optic disc is found one to two disc diameters nasal to the fovea, which lies at the centre of the macu-lar area.

Although micro-anatomical studies allow us to identify 13 or more layers in the fundus in depth, not all of these have ophthalmoscopic significance in the normal fundus. In abnormal fundi, however, an appreciation of the micro-anatomy helps to localize lesions in the depth of the fundus. Anatomical localization then contributes to the pathological diagnosis. The full details of the retina and fundus in depth are revealed in *Diagram 4*. The 10 identifiable retinal layers are: internal limiting membrane, nerve fibre layer, ganglion cell layer, inner plexiform layer, inner nuclear layer, outer plexiform layer, outer nuclear layer, external limiting membrane, rod and cone layer and the pigment epithelium. External to the retina is the choroid consisting of Bruch's membrane (an elastic and collagen tissue membrane), choriocapillaris with supporting arterial and venous systems, and finally the sclera, that is, the external coat of the eye.

From the ophthalmoscopic viewpoint not all of these layers have significance, but the appearances of the fundus are to some extent dependent on the age of the subject. What is the relationship of the retinal vessels to the retinal layers? The major branches of the retinal artery and vein run towards the retinal periphery from the disc, superficially, in the retinal nerve fibre layer (*Diagram 5*). Divisions of these vessels remain at this level until the pre-capillary divisions. Thereafter the vessels run at two levels, a superficial capillary net running also in the nerve fibre layer and a deep capillary net lying in

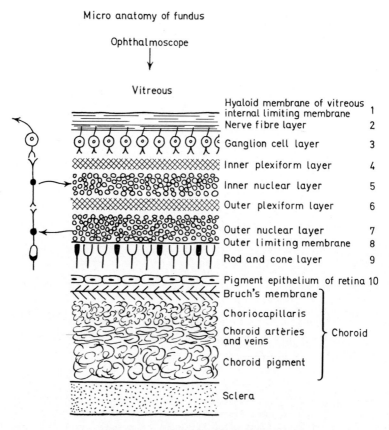

Micro anatomy of fundus

Ophthalmoscope

Vitreous

Hyaloid membrane of vitreous	
internal limiting membrane	1
Nerve fibre layer	2
Ganglion cell layer	3
Inner plexiform layer	4
Inner nuclear layer	5
Outer plexiform layer	6
Outer nuclear layer	7
Outer limiting membrane	8
Rod and cone layer	9
Pigment epithelium of retina	10
Bruch's membrane	
Choriocapillaris	
Choroid artèries and veins	Choroid
Choroid pigment	
Sclera	

Diagram 4. *Microanatomy of the fundus*

the boundary plane between the inner nuclear layer and the outer plexiform layer. There are connections between the two layers. Variations from this general pattern occur in the region of the optic nerve head and at the macula. In all retinal zones the retinal arteries are surrounded by a capillary-free zone of between 50 and 120 micrometres.

The region of the optic nerve head.—Here the capillary networks

10

are modified in that the superficial layer is more complex and runs at varying levels; three or four levels in all can be identified. Additionally, there are radial circumpapillary capillaries which seem to follow the nerve fibre pattern surrounding the disc. These capillaries run an irregular distance from the disc margin in the four quadrants of the retina.

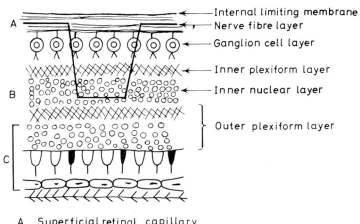

A   Superficial retinal capillary
    network

B   Deep retinal capillary
    network

C   Receive metabolites from
    choriocapillaris

Diagram 5. Retinal blood supply

In the macular area.—The fovea itself an area of 0·4 mm square is completely avascular.

In the extreme peripheral retina.—The deep capillary net gradually disappears.

Ophthalmoscopically significant layers

A superficial light reflex results from reflection of the ophthalmoscope light from the internal limiting membrane of the retina (*Diagram 6*). This gives a young person's retina a silken surface sheen. In the ageing retina, this appearance becomes much modified. A general appreciation of the nerve fibre layer may be gained in some fundi, the nerve fibres radiate from the optic nerve head in all directions, but with a preponderant inclination towards the temporal side of the retina, the greatest nerve fibre bulk supplying the macular area. In some normal fundi, nerve fibres are myelinated and appear brilliantly white, clearly identifying the nerve fibre pattern. Most commonly,

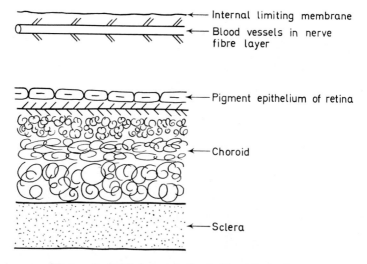

Diagram 6. Ophthalmoscopically significant fundus layers

myelination of retinal nerve fibres occurs in the optic disc area, but occasionally myelinated nerve fibres are seen more peripherally. The remaining layers of the retina, blood vessels apart, contribute little to the ophthalmoscopic view, although reflexes from the external limiting membrane may be evident in the younger subject. The pigment epithelium of the retina, its outermost layer, in contrast, contributes significantly to the ophthalmoscopic view of the fundus. The overall colour of the fundus is dependent on its degree of pigmentation (see Figures 2, 29, 45) as are views of the deeper layers of the fundus, that is, choroid and sclera. Thus, if the pigment layer of the retina is densely pigmented, the fundus appears correspondingly darker in colour and detail of choroidal structures is obscured. On the other hand, in a lightly pigmented pigment layer, the fundus appears much lighter red in colour and choroidal detail is correspondingly more visible. The other feature worth noting as contributory to the ophthalmoscopic view is the degree of pigmentation of the choroid. Its density will correspond to the pigmentation of the pigment layer of the retina. In general, the degree of pigmentation of a fundus is determined by hereditary, racial and metabolic factors (ability to produce melanin).

The region of the optic nerve head deserves special comment, for this region is open to considerable normal anatomical variation. An

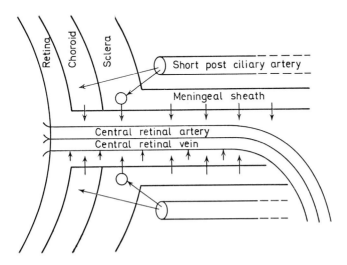

Diagram 7. Blood supply of optic nerve head

appreciation of these normal variations is a prerequisite to the recognition of abnormal features when they occur (*see Figures 1, 6, 7*). Two aspects must be considered, disc configuration and disc colour.

Refractive error (ametropia) considerably influences the configuration and overall size of the optic nerve head. For example, in myopia the optic disc is very large compared with the disc in a hypermetropia where the optic disc appears rather small. In the emmetropic eye, although the disc is generally circular in outline, irregularities may be present without affecting function. The contour of the optic disc is provided by the termination of the retinal and choroidal layers including their pigmentation, and the abrupt change in direction of the nerve fibres to a posterior direction to pass through the lamina cribrosa. Pigmentation in the choroid and the pigment layer of the retina may occasionally terminate some distance away from the true disc margins. In such cases the optic disc margin is less well demarcated. Absence of choroid and all layers but the nerve fibre layer of the retina, occurs in a crescentric fashion at the disc circumference. Crescents are a normal variation, occasionally they may totally surround the disc. Between the disc margin and the central pit-like area wherein the lamina cribrosa of the sclera is generally visible, is a region described as the rim of the optic nerve head. The rim is pinkish in colour, being composed of the nerve fibres and their attendant nutrient blood vessels. The nerve fibres are numerous and more crowded on the nasal aspects of the optic nerve head than on the temporal aspect, causing the nasal aspect of the normal optic disc to appear more highly coloured (pink) than the temporal aspect of the disc, that is, there is physiological temporal disc pallor. Considerable variation in the pattern of the retinal vessels contribute to variation in the appearance of the normal disc. Vascular malformations in this region are relatively common and embryonic remnants may also confuse the picture. The blood supply of the optic nerve head is illustrated in *Diagram 7*.

3—The Pathologic Fundus

The ways in which the fundus can respond to disease are limited. As a result, certain pathological fundus features may be common to many disorders. An example of this is the presence of microaneurysms in the retinal circulation in diabetic retinopathy, venous stasis retinopathy, the retinopathies of hyperviscosity syndromes, anaemia and several others. The very vascular nature of the fundus makes it likely that many disorders will have a circulatory origin. Although the pathogenesis of all retinopathies is not fully understood, vascular effects, whether primary or secondary, are readily identified as components of the presenting picture.

HAEMORRHAGE

Vitreous haemorrhage

Vitreous haemorrhage from retinal sources implies a defect in the hyaloid membrane, which, if intact, may contain even massive bleeding.

Vitreous haemorrhage may be total or subtotal. In the former case, the vitreous gel is saturated with blood and blood clot, totally obscuring any view of the fundus. The normal red glow of reflected light from the fundus seen ophthalmoscopically (the red reflex), is absent. Less than total vitreous haemorrhage is seen as strands, wisps or blobs of blood and blood clot or diffusely scattered red blood cells. All of these occurrences somewhat obscure the view of the fundus. Contrasting against the red reflex glow, small vitreous haemorrhages appear as black strands or wisps.

Subhyaloid haemorrhage

Subhyaloid haemorrhage refers to bleeding into the tissue plane between the internal limiting membrane of the retina and the hyaloid membrane of the vitreous. In this space the haemorrhage forms a sheet or pool which is limited anteriorly and posteriorly but not laterally. Blood, which does not clot in this situation, is influenced by gravity, the red cells tending to settle under its influence and to separate from the plasma. Within hours, the upper border of the haemorrhage is horizontal, showing this gravitational effect.

Haemorrhage into nerve fibre layer

Haemorrhages into the nerve fibre layer appear as linear, spindle shaped or flame shaped, that is, multilinear hacmorrhages. In this layer the free blood is confined by the radiating nerve fibres, accounting for the configuration of these haemorrhages. As we descend into the retina, haemorrhages in the inner, and less frequently the outer molecular layers of the retina, appear dot like, as the blood is confined by the cell bodies of the nerves which constitute these layers. In the plexiform layers of the retina the haemorrhages are a little more diffuse and appear blob like.

Subretinal haemorrhage is bleeding into the plane of cleavage between the rod and cone layer and the pigment epithelium layer, of the retina. Embryologically the potential space between these two layers represents the cavity between the two walls of the developing optic cup. Subretinal haemorrhage is therefore relatively poorly confined and seeps in all directions in a diffuse manner. These haemorrhages may cover large areas and have irregular expanding borders. If bleeding has been copious, rapid gravitational effects can be observed with changes in the patient's posture.

Haemorrhage beneath the pigment epithelial layer of the retina tends to be well confined, and is usually related to a rupture in the membrane of Bruch, which is normally adherent to it. The circumstances under which this membrane ruptures (trauma and pseudoxanthoma elasticum) tend to occasion the appearance of diffuse linear type haemorrhages of great extent.

Haemorrhage within the choroid has a relatively free ability to expand and forms pool-like areas whose ophthalmoscopic appearance is governed by the density of the overlying pigmentation. Generally, choroidal haemorrhages appear as dark reddish-blue areas, obviously deep in the fundus. Their appearance may be mistaken for that of a choroidal neoplasm. The fact that these haemorrhages absorb, leaving a normal fundus, is a clear distinguishing factor. Immediate differentiation is possible by fluorescein angiography.

EXUDATES

The term exudate should be reserved for retinal deposits resulting from the escape of plasma and white cells from defective blood vessels. Exudates may be classified into three subgroups: (1) oedema—of varying albumin or fibrin content; (2) lipid deposits; (3) cellular infiltration.

Oedema

Oedema is a feature of many retinopathies. When the albumin content is low, the oedema appears transparent but, as the albumin content rises, so the transparency decreases. In severe retinal oedema in hypertension, fibrin in the oedema may result in 'fusion' of the retinal layers.

Oedema of the macular region causes distortion of vision (metamorphopsia) and a reduction of image size due to separation of the light-sensitive elements. If persistent, macular oedema forms vacuoles in the retina with permanent interference with visual function.

Oedema of the optic nerve head causes a mushroom-like elevation of the optic disc anterior to the plane of the retina. Its causes are discussed later. This area of tissue is capable of great swelling without interference with function. Inflammatory oedema as opposed to the oedema of congestion is accompanied by loss of vision.

Lipid deposits

The currently held view is that lipid deposits in the retina represent the remains of plasma leakage from defective retinal vessels (see Figure 13). Fluorescein angiography demonstrates leaking blood vessels, for example, in relation to circinate lipid deposits (see Figure 13). Destruction of these vessels by photocoagulation is consequently followed by absorption of the lipid deposits.

Disposal of lipid remnants of plasma exudation is effected by histiocytes. Fat-laden histiocytes and microglia are seen in histological preparations of retinopathies manifesting lipid deposits. Cholesterol crystals are found in the 'harder' exudates giving them a glistening character. Rarely, calcification of lipid deposits may occur.

Cellular infiltration

Cellular infiltration occurs in inflammation of the choroid and retina, for example in tuberculosis, syphilis, toxoplasmosis and toxocariasis. The degree of accompanying plasma exudation depends on the activity of the lesion (see Figure 39), that is, size of lesion and the local vascular reaction. The affected area in a fundus may be obscured in the ophthalmoscopic view by showers of inflammatory cells in the vitreous adjacent to the active focus in the fundus. Pigment

17

dispersion is also a feature which becomes more evident as the inflammatory activity ceases.

TISSUE DEGENERATIONS

Tissue degenerations, like exudates, cause retinal deposits of a discrete or generalized nature. They may be classified into 7 categories. (1) Cotton wool patches; (2) Ischaemic necrosis of the retina; (3) Lipid degeneration of retinal ganglion cells; (4) Colloid bodies—drusen; (5) Tapeto-retinal degenerations; (6) Optic atrophy and choroidal atrophy; (7) Retinopathy of retinal detachment.

Cotton wool patches

Cotton wool patches, otherwise known as retinal soft exudates, are the local ischaemic response to closure of a retinal precapillary arteriole. The capillaries normally supplied by this arteriole remain patent but empty of blood, that is, they are not perfused. The overlying ganglion cells and nerve fibres undergo rapid degeneration. Histologically the characteristic finding in a cotton wool patch is the cytoid body, which is a terminal bulbous swelling of a nerve fibre. The precapillary arteriole shows cellular necrosis, the result of infiltration of its wall with hyaline lipoid material. Cotton wool patches are particularly found in hypertension, diabetes mellitus, septicaemia and severe anaemia (*see Plates and Figures 16, 23, 24*).

Ischaemic necrosis of the retina

Occlusion of the central retinal artery or one of its major branches gives rise to a milky opacification of the whole retina supplied by the affected vessel. This appearance is accounted for by cloudy swelling of the retinal ganglion cell layer with attendant oedema of the inner retinal layers (*see Figure 20*). The macula in this condition appears densely clouded but the fovea is relatively unaffected, leaving the red appearance of the choroid visible and contrasting at this site, which is known as the cherry-red spot.

Inherited metabolic disorders—the lipoidoses

The following examples of the lipoidoses are gangliosidosis and sphingomyelin lipoidosis.

Gangliosidosis (Tay–Sach's disease: Infantile amourotic family idiocy).—Accumulation of gangliosides causes disruption of retinal ganglion cells, giving rise to a picture not dissimilar to that of central retinal artery occlusion. The retina is milky white except for the cherry-red spot of the fovea.

Sphingomyelin lipoidosis (*Niemann–Pick disease*).—The ophthalmoscopic picture is of a foveal cherry-red spot surrounded by a milky opaque zone. Added to disruption of ganglion cells are oedema of the plexiform layers of the retina with deposits of characteristic foam cells.

Colloid bodies or drusen

Degeneration of collagen tissue on Bruch's membrane presents as yellowish spots, discrete or confluent. The diameter of individual bodies varies from pin-point to the equivalent diameter of a large retinal vessel. These bodies are usually associated with a corresponding defect in the overlying retinal pigment epithelium. They are found in a wide variety of normal and abnormal fundi; visual impairment is unusual. An exception to this is seen in the macular degeneration associated with massive central colloid bodies known as 'honeycomb choroiditis'.

Tapeto-retinal degenerations

Degeneration in the retinitis pigmentosa group of retinopathies may be (1) primary or (2) secondary to other retinal disease, for example, syphilis, rubella and measles.

Histologically, disappearance of the neuro-epithelium occurs with earliest affection of the rods (night blindness). The neural pigment epithelium is grossly affected with migration of pigment cells and aggregation of pigment often around blood vessels. In time, the external limiting membrane of the retina fuses with Bruch's membrane. Glial tissue proliferates in the worst affected areas. Retinal vessels are generally attenuated.

Optic atrophy and choroidal atrophy

Atrophy of the optic nerve secondary to retinal disease is termed secondary optic atrophy as opposed to intrinsic disease of the nerve, which is termed primary optic atrophy.

Histopathology of optic atrophy shows loss of axis cylinders of the nerve fibres, overgrowth of glia and connective tissue septae.

Choroidal atrophy may be generalized or localized and one form is given the term choroidal sclerosis. This implies a sclerotic degeneration of the choroidal arteries which accordingly produces atrophy of the choroidal tissue including the capillary layer and Bruch's membrane. The 'sclerosis' may be due to atherosclerosis, fatty necrosis or cellular infiltration.

Local or disseminated patches of choroidoretinal atrophy follow in the wake of local inflammatory disease (*see Figure 38*).

Retinopathy of retinal detachment

Primary retinal detachment implies a local retinal or vitreoretinal degeneration with perforation of the retina and escape of fluid into the subretinal space, that is, between rod and cone layer and the retinal pigment epithelium. This tissue plane is a natural one for separation to occur. Embryologically this represents the space between the inner and outer walls of the optic cup.

Another type of retinal degeneration results in a splitting of the retina at the level of the inner plexiform layer. The resultant loss of visual function is irreversible. The principal varieties of this degeneration are the juvenile hereditary and the senile forms. It is given the term retinoschisis and may appear as a shallow detachment or a cyst-like balloon detachment.

Secondary retinal detachment is the result of haemorrhage, exudate or tumour beneath the retina.

TISSUE FORMATION

The production of new tissue may be the result of (1) proliferation of retinal blood vessels; (2) proliferation of retinal pigment epithelium; (3) neoplasia.

Proliferation of retinal blood vessels

The appearance and growth of new retinal vessels occurs in pathological circumstances. Diabetic retinopathy, venous occlusive retinopathy and the retinopathy of prematurity (retrolental fibroplasia) are examples of the incidence of retinal neovascularization. Newly-formed retinal vessels may be intraretinal, preretinal, subretinal, on the optic nerve head, or intramural. (*See Figures 21, 25, 26, 36.*)

Until the time when a vasoformative factor is identified in pathological retinas, the only known common factor to retinopathies supporting new retinal vessels is tissue anoxia. While there is abundant experimental proof of the role of anoxia in stimulating new vessel growth it is not yet possible to indict anoxia as the definite cause, in all instances, of neovascularization in the retina.

Intraretinal, preretinal (including intravitreal) and optic nerve head new vessels are the major problem in the visually crippling condition of diabetic retinopathy. The tendency of new vessels to rupture and bleed, makes their control imperative if sight is to be maintained.

Subretinal new vessels constitute a minor phenomenon, being mainly found in post-inflammatory or degenerative lesions, usually of a local nature. Anastomoses with choroidal vessels can occur. Recanalization of thrombosed retinal veins by the development of intramural new vessels, unfortunately does not lead to restoration of retinal function.

Proliferation of retinal pigment epithelium

The causative factor may be (1) hyperplasia of the retinal pigment epithelium or (2) fundus flavimaculatus.

Hyperplasia of the retinal pigment epithelium occurs in the region of the optic nerve head, but is associated with more peripheral pigment regeneration. It is an entirely benign condition, but it may be confused in diagnosis with a malignant choroidal tumour.

Fundus flavimaculatus presents as white or yellowish fleck-like lesions, sometimes described as fish-tail in shape, which are scattered over the posterior fundus. These lesions may be mistaken for colloid bodies but they are the product of the retinal pigment epithelium. An acid mucopolysaccharide is thought to be elaborated by pigment epithelium cells.

Neoplasia

Neoplasia may occur (1) in the choroid, as angioma, benign melanoma, malignant melanoma or secondary tumours; (2) in the retina as angioma, glioma (retinoblastoma) or malignant melanoma of retinal pigment epithelium; (3) in the optic nerve as primary glioma, primary meningioma, melanocytoma or secondary tumour.

Choroidal angiomas.—Angiomas of the choroid present as fundus tumours which are easily and often mistaken for a malignant melanoma. Fluorescence angiography provides a satisfactory means of diagnosis. The lesion is capable of expansion and is accompanied by exudative phenomena which cause loss of vision.

Benign melanoma.—The borderline between a benign and a malignant melanoma may be hard to determine especially as the former may undergo malignant change (*see Figure 45*).

Malignant melanoma (*see* page 136).

Secondary tumours (*see* page 138).

Retina.—Angioma—(*see* page 140).

Glioma (retinoblastoma) is a malignant tumour which spreads by local growth and beyond by metastases. A tumour of infancy and childhood amenable to treatment by radiotherapy. It is the most serious concern in the differential diagnosis of a retrolental white mass seen in a child's eye.

Malignant melanoma of the retinal pigment epithelium is a histopathological diagnosis. Clinically, these rare tumours behave as malignant melanomas of the choroid (*see* page 136).

Optic nerve.—The ophthalmoscopic signs of glioma and meningioma depend on the location of the tumour in the nerve. The signs are unilateral, with proprosis papilloedema and optic atrophy the principal effects.

Secondary tumours in the optic nerve are very rare.

4—Fluorescein Angiography

Appreciation of ophthalmoscopic features in the fundus in systemic and ocular disorders has been greatly increased since the advent of fluorescein angiography.

The concept of fluorescein angiography was introduced in 1960/61 by Novotny and Alvis, in America, following attempts to study circulation times by utilizing intravascular dyes. The logic of this technique is that retinal blood vessels can be illuminated by the presence in them of a fluorescent dye. The fluorescent vessels are photographed in order to obtain the angiogram. The dye used is sodium fluorescein and it is introduced into the circulation by intravenous injection, via the cubital vein. The dye is introduced in a small quantity, 3 ml of high concentration (25 per cent). The dye passes through the venous system to enter the right side of the heart, then passes through the pulmonary circulation to be pumped out into the systemic arterial system by the left ventricle. Fractions of the dye stream pass into all the major arteries and thus the eye receives the dye via the internal carotid and the ophthalmic arteries. The dye thence passes into the fundus (1) through the central retinal artery and (2) into the choroid through the short posterior ciliary arteries. Normal retinal blood vessels, that is, arteries, capillaries and veins are impermeable to the dye, which, after circulating through the retinal circulation, passes back into the systemic circulation to become diluted and eventually recirculated in much lower concentration. The fact that vessels in the retinal circulation are impervious to the dye is one of the key factors in the success of this technique. Most capillary circulations elsewhere in the body do not retain the dye, which rapidly stains most body tissues. The dye loosely binds to serum albumin but is fairly rapidly excreted from the body, mainly in the urine.

There are generally no ill effects from the injection from this dye, only 5 per cent of patients complaining of a very transient nausea. The dye colours the whole body skin a yellowish colour, which persists for up to 6 hours. The bulk of the dye is passed in the urine in the first few hours after injection, and the majority of the dye has left the body within 24 hours. Traces are, however, eliminated over the next few days. This is an important point to note, for the presence of the fluorescein in body fluids, even in small quantities, can upset biochemical assays which are performed by fluorescent spectroscopy.

Following the intravenous injection of a small quantity of fluorescein dye, its arrival in the retinal circulation in a normal patient at rest can be observed after an interval of some 10–15 seconds. Its passage through the retinal circulation occupies approximately a further 10 seconds, and its re-circulation occurs some 25–30 seconds later. The information which can be derived from this technique involves a study of the passage of the dye through the retinal and choroidal circulations on the initial dye transit. Thereafter, successive studies at intervals up to 10–15 minutes after the injection of the dye also may yield valuable information. Photographs are accordingly taken during the initial dye transit at intervals of 1 second or less. Following this, photographs are taken at intervals of 1 minute for the remaining period.

The passage of the dye fluorescein through the fundus circulations can only be viewed by inducing the dye to fluoresce. This is achieved by illumination of the fundus with a blue light of the appropriate wavelength, that is, about 475 nm. Light of this wavelength is absorbed by the dye and is then re-emitted as a greenish light of wavelength around 520 nm. Thus the retinal vessels when so viewed appear in brilliant fluorescent green, contrasting with the blue background. The phenomenon can be viewed by a suitably modified ophthalmoscope. This requires incorporation of a blue filter and a raising of the normal level of illumination. The phenomena, however, that are viewed are *very transient*, and worthwhile information is difficult to gain from this type of observation by ophthalmoscopy. *It is therefore necessary to photograph the sequence of events.* Angiograms are obtained by selectively recording the emitted greenish fluorescent light, with the elimination of all other light from the record. This is achieved by placing a green filter in front of the film in the fundus camera, the filter having the characteristic that it passes only the green fluorescent light reaching it from the fundus and that it absorbs or reflects the reflected blue light from the fundus (*Diagram 8*). The film material used to record the sequence of events is a high quality conventional monochrome film and is so processed that a moderately high-contrast image results. Full details of the technique of fluorescein angiography can be found in *Fluorescence Photography of the Eye.**

In order to derive the utmost benefit from the illustrations it will be necessary for the student to appreciate the basic points of interpretation of fluorescein angiograms.

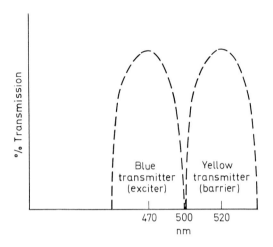

Diagram 8. Filters for fluorescein angiography

Normal phenomena

The presence of the fluorescein in the angiograms in this book is denoted by the white areas in the photographs, the absence of the fluorescein being denoted by the black areas. The retinal circulation is depicted in the foreground; the choroidal circulation is depicted in the background (*Diagram 9*). Owing to the normal anatomical arrangement of the fundus layers (*see Diagram 4*) the choroidal flow of fluorescein dye is more or less viewed as a background fluorescent glow. The glow commences with choroidal arterial filling, but the overlying choroidal capillary bed soon masks any detail of the larger choroidal vessels. The view of the choroidal circulation is dependent upon the degree of pigmentation of the overlying retinal pigment epithelium. The retinal circulation, unlike the choroid which is viewed end on (*Diagram 9*), is seen at 90 degrees to the axis of view. Retinal arterial filling occurs very rapidly, all the retinal arteries

* Rosen, E. S. (1969). London; Butterworths.

being filled within 1 second of dye appearance in the central retinal artery. The detail and view of the retinal capillary circulation is limited by the fluorescent glow from the background. If this is somewhat masked by dense pigmentation in the retinal pigment epithelium, the retinal capillary circulation may achieve complete definition. Retinal vein filling has a characteristic striped appearance,

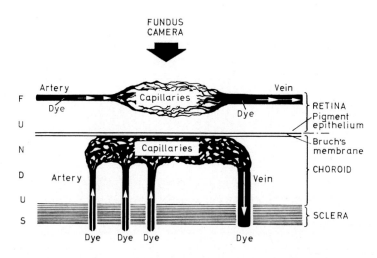

Diagram 9. Development of fluorescein in choroid and retina. Angiographic significant layers

owing to the laminar flow or streaming of fluorescein in normal healthy retinal vessels. As dye columns enter a vein from its tributaries, so the streaming appearance is produced; the columns of dye gradually coalesce to give an even fluorescence of the retinal vein at the latter part of the dye transit. The circulation in the optic nerve head has several components, principally derived from choroidal supply, but often obscured by retinal venous tributaries. Thus, its circulation may or may not be easy to define. Observations are necessary from the earliest appearance of the dye in the eye.

Unlike the retina, where dye does not escape from vessels, the choroid shows extravascular space staining with dye as it penetrates the walls of the choroidal capillary bed. There is a rapid interchange of intravascular and extravascular tissue fluid in the choroid, and thus the dye is rapidly cleared from extravascular choroidal tissue. The sclera, however, lying behind the choroid and containing a great deal of collagen, easily stains with fluorescein, which gains access to it from the extravascular spaces of the choroid initially, and later by seepage through the scleral wall from the orbital aspects of the eye. Many minutes after the dye has initially circulated through the eye, its intravascular concentration has fallen greatly as it has become diluted with and distributed throughout the body fluids, before elimination through the kidney. At this stage, the retinal and choroidal blood vessels are no longer fluorescent, but scleral fluorescence, appearing within minutes of the injection, persists for an hour or two, and provides the fluorescent backcloth to the whole of the fundus. The visibility of this backcloth is dependent upon the degree of pigmentation of the fundus, that is, in the retinal pigment epithelium and the choroid. Where pigmentation is deficient, then a fluorescent glow from the sclera silhouettes all the layers anterior to it. The normal tissues of the optic disc, principally the lamina cribrosa, also fluoresce in this later phase of the photographic sequence.

So much for normal phenomena, although it is strongly recommended that the student studies a normal sequence of fluorescein angiograms in order to become fully acquainted with normal appearances. For this he is again referred to *Fluorescence Photography of the Eye*.

Some pathological phenomena seen in fluorescein angiograms

(1) Abnormalities of blood flow in both retinal and choroidal circulations can be demonstrated by fluorescein angiography, thus regional slowing of the circulation or failure of the circulation can be depicted (for example, *Figures 19, 20*).

(2) The retinal circulation in some pathological circumstances becomes permeable to the dye, this being known as dye leakage (*see Figures 8, 14C, 36*).

(3) As a result of dye leakage, tissue staining with the fluorescein will occur. This includes the staining of inflammatory exudate (*see Figure 37*), scar tissue (*see Figure 39*) and the staining of vessel walls (*see Figure 27*).

(4) Pigmentary faults in the fundus, especially in the retinal pigment epithelium, are brilliantly demonstrated. Absence of pigment or migration of pigment from the retinal epithelium, generally or locally, provides a 'window' on choroidal fluorescent phenomena (*see Figures 38, 44*). Conversely, pigmentary aggregates at this level provide a mask over choroidal fluorescent phenomena (*see Figure 45*).

(5) Haemorrhage in the retina or choroid is always non-fluorescent, and appears black. If the haemorrhage is superficial it will mask

all underlying fluorescent features (*see Figure 30*). If the haemorrhage is deep, overlying fluorescent features will contrast significantly (*see Figure 41*).

(6) Oedema exudates will stain with fluorescein, especially if they contain albumin (*see Figures 17, 33*). Lipid deposits are entirely non-fluorescent (*see Figure 13*).

(7) In tissue degeneration, cotton wool patches are characterized by the non-perfused retinal capillaries beneath the patch (*see Figure 23*); dilated capillaries surround the patch which itself becomes fluorescent in time (*see Figure 17*).

(8) Neovascularization in the retina is readily identified by consistent dye leakage (*see Figures 21, 27, 36*).

SECTION II

Colour Plates

The sequence numbers of the plates in this section pair with those of the Monographs in Section III and, therefore with the angiograms reproduced in that section.

References to the colour plates appear in the paragraphs headed Ophthalmoscopic Findings. Those to the corresponding angiograms, which, however, embrace larger fields, appear after the heading Fluorescein Angiograms

Colour Transparencies

Sets of mounted colour transparencies duplicated from the originals of these colour plates are available as an extra facility for the student and lecturer—*see* announcement on page ix.

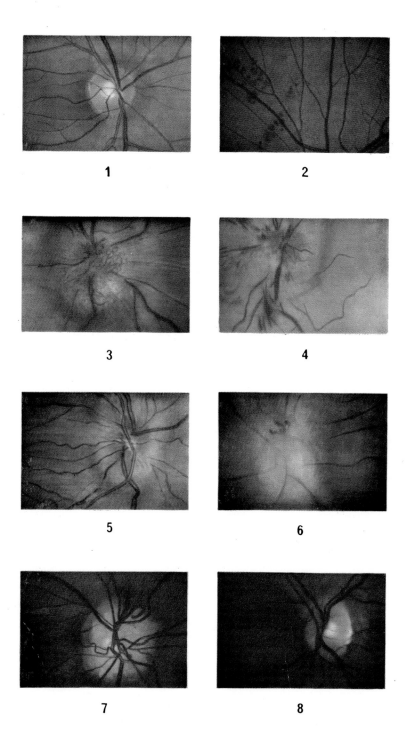

1

2

3

4

5

6

7

8

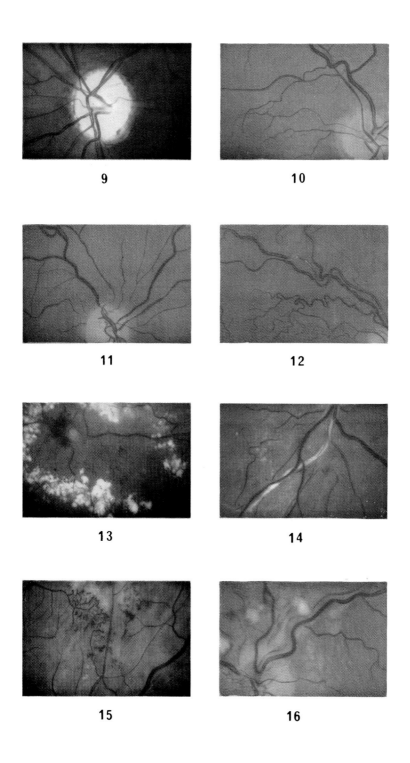

9

10

11

12

13

14

15

16

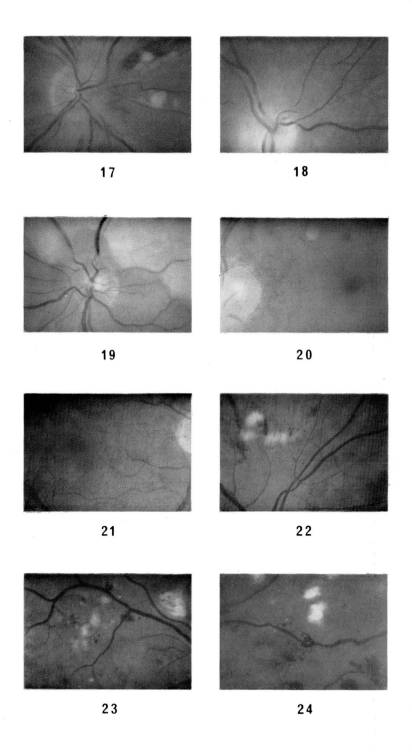

17

18

19

20

21

22

23

24

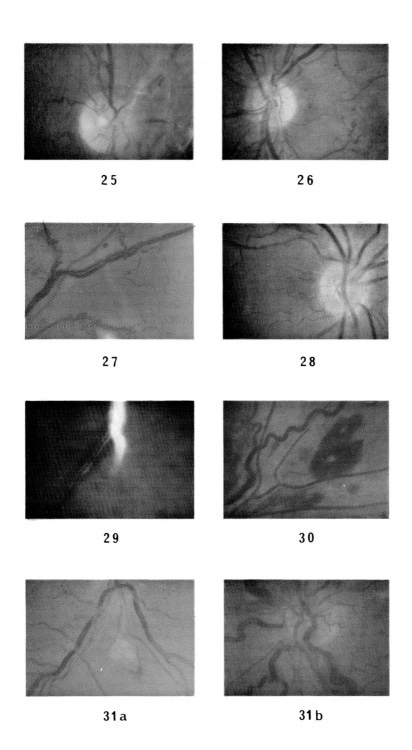

25

26

27

28

29

30

31 a

31 b

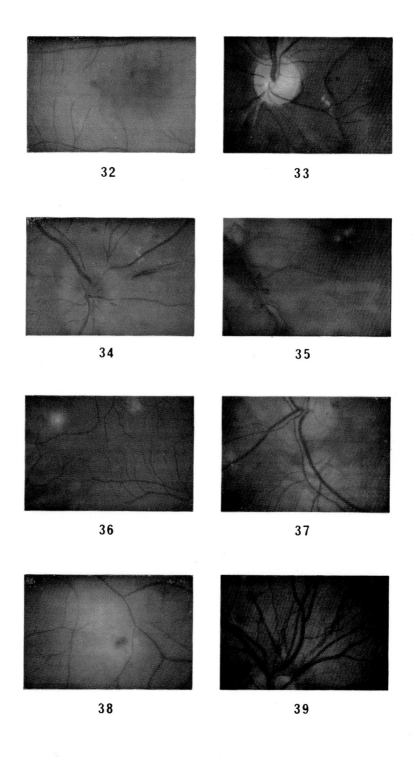

32

33

34

35

36

37

38

39

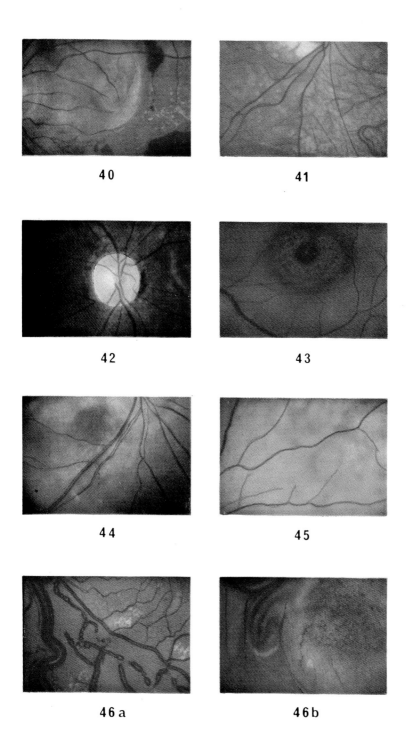

40

41

42

43

44

45

46 a

46 b

SECTION III

Ophthalmoscopic Findings in Systemic Disorders

1—Normal Fundus

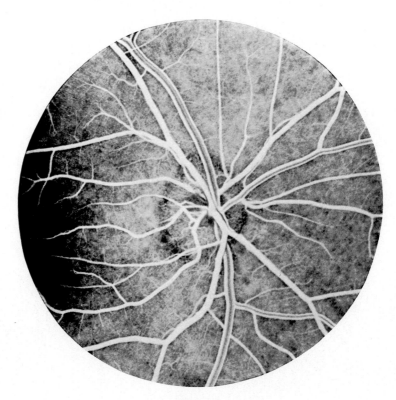

Figure 1

Clinical presentation: White woman aged 35 years.

Ocular features: Visual acuity 6/5 in each eye. Emmetropia.

Ophthalmoscopic findings: The region of the right optic disc (*Plate 1*) is illustrated especially for comparison with abnormal optic discs shown elsewhere in this book. The features to be noted are, the generally circular outline of the disc which clearly demarcates it from the adjacent fundus, and a central pale area from which the central retinal vessels and their branches emerge. A stereoscopic view showed that this central pale area is a small pit which is known as the physiological optic cup. This is normal optic disc configuration. Between the margins of the central physiological optic cup and the outer margin of the optic disc is a wide rim of pinkish tissue, which is of greater density on the nasal aspect of the nerve head. The rim is composed of retinal nerve fibres which course centripetally across the retinal surface and dip down into the optic nerve proper. The nerve fibres accompanied by their nutrient blood vessels are more densely aggregated on the nasal side of the optic nerve head, accounting for the nasal and temporal colour disparity.

Fluorescein angiogram: An angiogram of a normal optic disc and surrounding fundus is shown in *Figure 1*. Taken in the mid-venous phase of dye circulation, it illustrates both choroidal fluorescence in the background and retinal vessel fluorescence in the foreground. Additionally, the capillaries of the disc circulation are demonstrated. The central retinal artery bifurcates immediately on entering the retina, into an upper and lower branch, which in turn divide into temporal and nasal branches. The central retinal vein main branches receive corresponding tributaries. Apart from retinal venous tributaries crossing its surface, the blood supply of the optic disc is derived from choroidal and posterior ciliary circulations. Towards the macular area, on the left of the picture, the fall-off in fluorescent intensity is indicative of the increasing pigmentation of this area. Examples are shown later where this pigmentation is disrupted.

2—Normal Fundus containing Pigmentary Variation

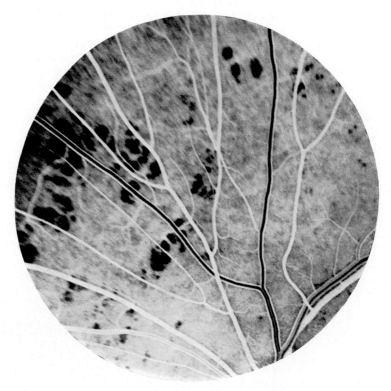

Figure 2

Clinical presentation: White man aged 25 years.

Ocular features: Visual acuity 6/5 in each eye.

Ophthalmoscopic findings: Scattered cats-paw pigmentation was seen in both fundi. The zone illustrated (*Plate 2*) is above the right optic disc. The name of the pigmentation is self-descriptive.

Fluorescein angiogram: Early venous phase (*Figure 2*). The choroid is fully fluorescent at this stage and the abnormal pigmentation, being situated in the retinal pigment epithelium, is silhouetted against the underlying choroidal fluorescence. The cats-paw pigmentation represents a normal variation, and is due to localized proliferation and hyperpigmentation of the retinal pigment epithelium.

Additional notes: Fundus pigmentation of this type is referred to in the literature variously as 'grouped melanosis', 'bear-print pigmentation', or 'cats-paw pigmentation'.

3—*Acoustic Neuroma with Raised Intracranial Pressure*

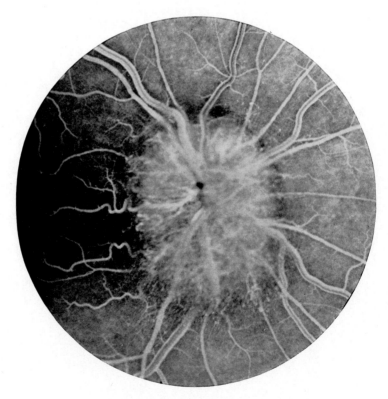

Figure 3

Clinical presentation: White man aged 45 years.

Systemic features: Six-month history of tinnitus, perceptual deafness on the left side and dizziness. Later symptoms included headache.

Ocular features: Visual acuity was unimpaired but the patient had unequivocal bilateral papilloedema.

Ophthalmoscopic findings: The right optic disc region is illustrated (*Plate 3*). There is gross swelling of the optic nerve head, with marked congestion of the retinal veins. The physiological optic cup is filled in and the disc may be described as having a woolly hyperaemic appearance. There were a few linear haemorrhages but no exudates.

Fluorescein angiogram: In the early phase of dye circulation illustrated, the most striking feature is the gross dilatation and possible proliferation of the capillary circulation in the optic nerve head (*Figure 3*). Angiography clearly demonstrates these vessels. Their congestion spreads beyond the disc margin and some radial retinal capillaries are also dilated, some with microaneurysmal dilatations.

Their incontinence to fluorescein was rapidly demonstrated as the dye leaked through the capillary walls and stained both the optic nerve head and the adjacent retina. Thus, in late phase the optic nerve head and surrounding retina well beyond the disc margins, had a persistent diffuse fluorescence.

This staining of the optic nerve head with the fluorescein is a characteristic finding in papilloedema and is a major sign which differentiates true papilloedema from pseudo-papilloedema.

Additional clinical note: Following surgical removal of the acoustic neuroma, this patient returned to normal health and the optic disc appearances reverted to normal, his visual functions being unimpaired.

Optic disc elevation: see page 143.

4—Hodgkin's Disease

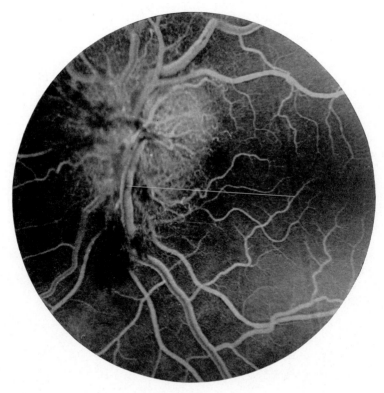

Figure 4

Clinical presentation: White man aged 53 years.

Systemic features: Anorexia, lassitude and weight loss. Examination revealed firm and rubbery enlargement of cervical and axillary lymph nodes. Despite therapy the patient's condition deteriorated over a four-month period and he developed progressive mediastinal involvement, with signs of superior vena cava obstruction.

Ocular symptoms: In the latter part of the clinical course of the disease vision in the left eye began to deteriorate.

Ophthalmoscopic findings: Gross papilloedema in the left eye with swelling of the optic disc, superficial disc haemorrhages and radiating flame-shaped haemorrhages beyond the disc margin (*Plate 4*). Loss of the physiological pit of the disc and engorgement of the retinal veins.

Fluorescein angiogram: The main component of the papilloedema is seen to be engorgement and dilatation of the capillaries of the optic nerve head (*Figure 4*). The radial circumpapillary retinal capillaries are dilated well beyond the disc margins in all quadrants. Engorgement of the retinal veins is seen in this mid-venous angiogram and the haemorrhages contrast against the underlying fluorescence.

Additional notes: There are no characteristic fundus changes in this disease and retinal complications are rare. They would tend to occur as a result of concomitant anaemia and thrombocytopenia.

The superior vena cava obstruction in this patient was considered to be a causative factor in the appearance of papilloedema.

5—Endocrine Exophthalmos

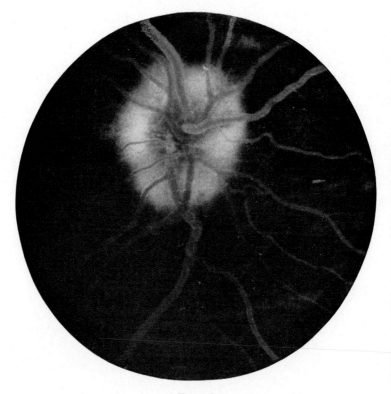

Figure 5

Clinical presentation: White woman aged 44 years.

Systemic features: Patient developed progressive exophthalmos following treatment of thyrotoxicosis. The degree of exophthalmos was such that she had difficulty in closing her eyelids and the conjunctiva was both congested and oedematous. She suffered diplopia as a result of extraocular muscle involvement in the exophthalmic process.

Ocular features: Apart from diplopia she had noted deterioration of vision, especially in her right eye, in recent weeks.

Ophthalmoscopic findings: There was asymmetrical but marked elevation of both optic nerve heads, the right (*Plate 5*) being more severe than the left. Additionally, both fundi revealed a horizontal pattern of choroidoretinal folds. These were the result of indentation of the globe by the engorged orbital contents.

Fluorescein angiogram: The engorgement and dilatation of the capillaries on the optic nerve head were the principal feature (*Figure 5*). These capillaries were incontinent to fluorescein, which stained both the optic nerve head and the surrounding retina vividly, for a period of hours. The stress lines or folds in the choroid and retina, the result of orbital indentation of the globe, are visible in the angiogram.
    This is true papilloedema but is the result of raised intra-orbital pressure as opposed to raised intracranial pressure.

Additional notes: Raised intra-orbital pressure obstructs venous outflow from the eye. The initial appearance of papilloedema, if untreated, is eventually superseded by optic atrophy. It is a sign indicating that orbital decompression should be performed without delay.

6—Sarcoidosis with Papilloedema

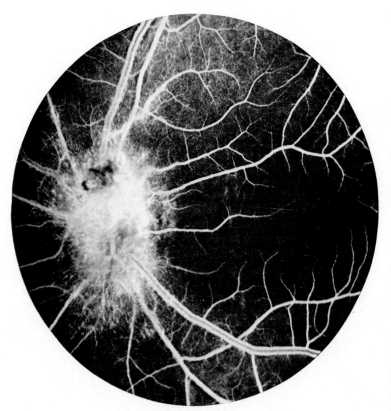

Figure 6

Clinical presentation: Negro (West Indian), woman aged 51 years.

Systemic features: This patient has suffered from a transitory skin eruption over the chest for the past $1\frac{1}{2}$ years. Additionally, dizziness, numbness of the right lower lip and diminished triceps and ankle jerks were noticed.

Laboratory investigations revealed an ESR of 45 mm in the first hour (Westergren) and slight hyperglobulinaemia. The Kveim test was positive. Treatment with steroids improved the symptoms.

Ocular symptoms: On examination, a chronic papilloedema of the left eye was found in 1969. This condition did not change much during the follow-up.

A transient swelling of the right disc was noticed several months ago. The patient's vision and visual fields remain normal.

Ophthalmoscopic findings: Ophthalmoscopy revealed a chronic papilloedema of the left eye (*Plate 6*). The disc margins are blurred with sheathing of the veins; flame-shaped haemorrhages on the upper disc margins are seen surrounded by oedema giving the 'out of focus' impression.

Fluorescein angiogram: A picture from the venous phase is illustrated in *Figure 6*. The disc margin is blurred all around with capillary engorgement. The physiological cup is not seen because of the swelling and dye leakage from the capillaries which are well defined. On the upper disc margin haemorrhages are seen as black spots. The whole disc is out of focus in comparison with the sharp picture of the macula and temporal retina, indicating the degree of swelling.

Additional notes: Sarcoidosis, also known as Besnier–Boeck–Schaumann disease, is a systemic disease of unknown cause. The disease involves lymph nodes, lungs, skin, eyes, liver, spleen, phalangeal bones and the nervous system. The histological features are quite pathognomonic—epithelioid cell tubercles with little necrosis. The tuberculin test is usually negative. Hyperglobulinaemia and leucopenia are common laboratory findings.

The diagnosis is based on the clinical picture, the Quinn test, the Kveim test and biopsy of an affected lymph node.

The most common ocular manifestation is an anterior uveitis (in about 44 per cent of the cases), choroiditis is less common. Perivasculitis retinae or involvement of the optic nerve head are also seen, the latter causing the picture of longstanding papilloedema.

7—Pseudopapilloedema: Drusen and Vascular Anomaly

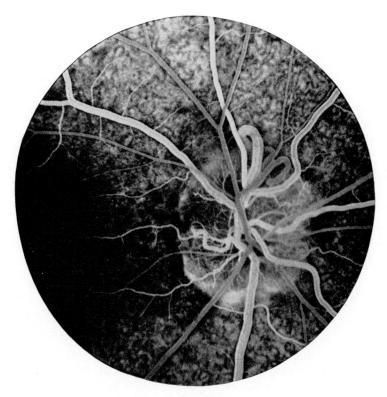

Figure 7

Clinical presentation: White boy aged 16 years.

Systemic features: Complaint of non-specific headaches for several weeks. There were no abnormal neurological signs.

Ocular features: There were no ocular symptoms, but both optic discs were found to be swollen and a diagnosis of papilloedema secondary to raised intracranial pressure was tentatively made. Radiographic studies of the skull failed to reveal any abnormality.

Ophthalmoscopic features: The right optic disc is illustrated in *Plate 7*. This disc is most unusual in appearance, being much larger than normal. It has an irregular outline and is quite grossly swollen. Apart from the blood vessels on its surface it is generally pale, and seems to contain irregular refractile bodies. The retinal vessels at first sight appear to be engorged, especially the veins. There is no physiological optic cup.

Fluorescein angiogram: The venous phase angiogram (*Figure 7*) shows most of the disc features. The retinal veins are of normal calibre, but the supranasal branch of both retinal vein and artery contain abnormal loops. Otherwise the vessels are normal. In the background the irregularity and swelling of the disc can be seen by the in-focus and out-of-focus appearance of different portions of the disc. This is an appearance characteristic of drusen or colloid bodies in the optic nerve head. These bodies slowly imbibe fluorescein and in late phase give a glistening irregular lumpy fluorescent appearance to the optic disc.

Additional notes: The diagnosis here is of pseudopapilloedema and the clinical diagnosis of true papilloedema the result of raised intra-cranial pressure, was incorrect. Both the vascular anomaly and the buried drusen in the optic nerve head which contributed to the disc swelling and its irregular appearance, often give rise to the mistaken diagnosis of papilloedema. Consequently a patient may be subjected to full neurological investigation without real need.

Diagnosis of buried drusen as a cause of pseudopapilloedema is supported by the clinical findings of a hard amorphous appearance of the disc elevations, irregular elevated disc margins and the presence of drusen in the other eye or in the eyes of members of the same family.

A non-congested, irregularly elevated optic disc, absence of physiologic cup and no pathologic alteration in the blood vessels should always suggest a diagnosis of pseudopapilloedema. Fluorescein angiographic studies can confirm normality of the blood vessels and can identify buried drusen by their late phase-irregular fluorescence.

51

8—*Multiple Sclerosis (Acute Retrobulbar Neuritis)*

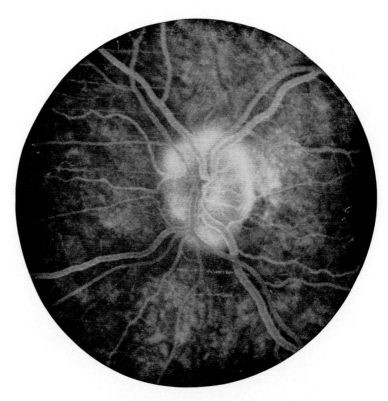

Figure 8

Clinical presentation: White woman aged 22 years.

Systemic features: Paraesthesiae in fingers of both hands.

Ocular features: The patient presented 4 days after the onset of blurring of vision in the left eye. Visual acuity was 6/60, visual field testing revealed a dense central scotoma. She complained of pain on moving the eye which was also tender to palpation. The vision gradually returned to 6/6 over a period of 84 days.

Ophthalmoscopic features: In the left optic disc, retinal blood vessels and fundus appeared normal at all times during the course of this disease. The left optic disc region is illustrated in *Plate 8* and it is emphasized that there is *no* swelling of this optic disc.

Fluorescein angiogram: The angiogram illustrated (*Figure 8*) was taken 11 days after onset of symptoms and is of the left optic disc region, 5 minutes after injection of dye. There had been a diffuse leakage of fluorescein from the optic disc, especially around its nasal circumference and the dye had diffused out into the nasal retina.

The incontinence of the optic disc capillaries for fluorescein in this case of acute retrobulbar neuritis reveals a phenomenon which could be termed 'sub-clinical papilloedema'. That is, there is no clinical evidence of disc swelling or inflammation, but the extremely sensitive fluorescein angiographic test revealed vascular features which could not be demonstrated in any other way. Serial angiography of this patient's eye was carried out at intervals over a period of 84 days, and the leakage of fluorescein gradually diminished until there was none. The reduction of dye leakage during the period corresponded with an improvement in visual acuity.

Optic disc elevation: Discussion, page 143.

9—Post-traumatic Optic Atrophy

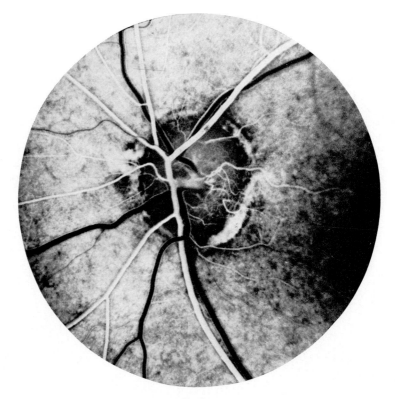

Figure 9

Clinical presentation: White woman aged 22 years.

Systemic features: The patient received head injuries in a road traffic accident 2 years previously. She sustained loss of sight in the left eye at the time of injury but otherwise made full recovery.

Ocular symptoms: Loss of sight in the left eye at the time of the accident with no subsequent recovery.

Ophthalmoscopic findings: A normal fundus except for gross optic atrophy. The disc is well demarcated and is flat (*Plate 9*).

Fluorescein angiogram: Early venous phase (*Figure 9*). The retinal vessels are normal, the arteries appearing a fluorescent white at this stage. Early laminar flow of dye can be seen in all veins as the dye enters from the venous tributaries. Background choroidal fluorescence is well developed and yet the optic disc contains little fluorescein. Its blood vessels have disappeared during the course of development of the optic atrophy. A few fluorescent minor branches of the retinal arteries and veins course across the disc surface.

Additional notes: Optic atrophy, loss of visual function associated with pallor of the optic disc, develops as a result of retinal disease with destruction of ganglion cells, optic nerve head disorders, for example, 'papillitis', papilloedema, glaucoma and finally, as a result of disease affecting the optic nerve, chiasma and optic tract (retrograde degeneration). Co-existence of optic atrophy in one eye with papilloedema in the other eye may be due to a sphenoidal ridge meningioma—the Foster Kennedy syndrome. Slow compression of one optic nerve resulting in optic atrophy and gradual involvement of the optic nerve of the other side gives initial papilloedema which also will progress to optic atrophy if the meningioma is left untreated.

A similar picture of unilateral optic atrophy with contralateral papilloedema is also connected with a diagnosis of ischaemic optic neuropathy often associated with the condition of giant cell (temporal) arteritis. Here the cause is primary ischaemic disease rather than the optic nerve compression found in the true Foster Kennedy syndrome.

10—Arteriosclerosis

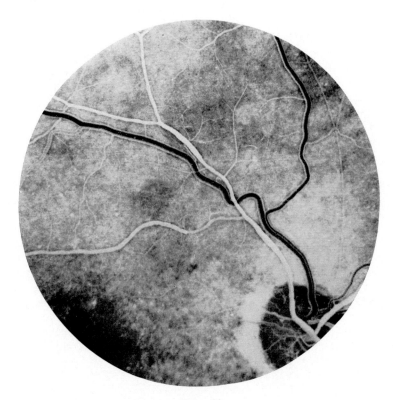

Figure 10

Clinical presentation: White man aged 58 years.

Systemic features: Two-year history of angina pectoris. Blood pressure = 200/100.

Ocular symptoms: Six-month history of failing vision. Right 6/24; left 6/36.

Ophthalmoscopic findings: Bilateral optic atrophy and gross irregularity of the retinal arteries. The superior temporal retinal artery illustrated in *Plate 10*, shows wall sheathing in the region of the optic disc and thereafter continuous calibre variations. Segments of relatively normal artery are preceded and succeeded by narrowed portions. This vessel has a silver-wire reflex.

Fluorescein angiogram: The pathological changes in the wall of the artery are reflected by the calibre of the vessel lumen, which is illustrated in this angiogram (*Figure 10*). The features represent the result of normal ageing processes or involutionary sclerosis, in retinal arteries. Added to this are the effects of a sustained hypertension. The ability of ageing arteries to respond to increased blood pressure is limited by the loss of elasticity of the vessel wall and fibrosis rather than hypertonus is the main cause of arterial narrowing.

The systolic type of hypertension from which this man suffers, blood pressure 200/100, is the result of generalized or systemic sclerotic changes in the major arteries of the body.

Senile arteriosclerosis

Arteriosclerosis is an involutionary change occurring in blood vessels of people generally over the age of 60 years. These changes affect vessels of the fundus.

The ophthalmoscopic picture reveals straightened arteries with a narrowed lumen. The arteries are pale, their reflex is less brilliant, the branching is more acute and some calibre variation may be detected. The veins are narrowed, and have a reduced axial reflex. At arteriovenous crossings no changes are seen.

Choroidal vessels can be affected, causing peripheral choroidal degeneration, pigmentary disturbances and colloid bodies.

If atherosclerosis with raised cholesterol levels is present, central retinal artery occlusion may follow, and bright shining plaques around and in the arteries can be found.

11—Hypertension

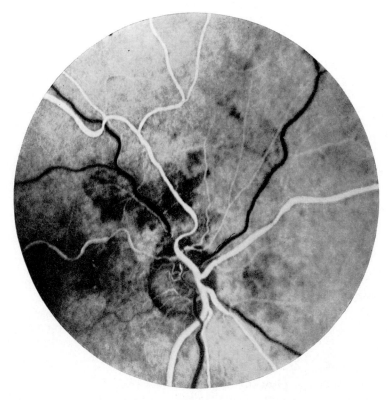

Figure 11

Clinical presentation: White man aged 58 years.

Systemic features: Five-year history of hypertension, angina pectoris and increasing dyspnoea on exertion. Blood pressure 210/100.

Ocular symptoms: Sudden loss of vision in the right eye one month previous to this examination. The vision had not recovered. His visual acuity was hand movements only and there was more or less total loss of the inferior visual field.

Ophthalmoscopic findings: Optic atrophy was striking as were the calibre variations in the superior branches of the central retinal artery (*Plate 11*). Gross narrowing of retinal arteries near the disc was accompanied by a thickening of the vessel wall. These appearances are consistent with retinal arterial occlusive disease most commonly seen in older hypertensive patients.

Fluorescein angiogram: Retinal arterial phase (*Figure 11*). Choroidal perfusion is not yet quite complete accounting for the non-fluorescent patches in the background of this photograph. The irregularities in the upper branches of the central retinal artery are demonstrated. It should be noted that the calibre of the arterial lumen appears wider than in the colour photograph; this is because by ophthalmoscopy and colour photography the red blood cell column in a vessel is seen and recorded, whereas in fluorescein angiography a fluorescent plasma column is recorded. In retinal vessels a central column of red blood cells is flanked by a cell-free plasma zone. Proximal arterial narrowing is succeeded by distal arterial dilatation.

12—Hypertension

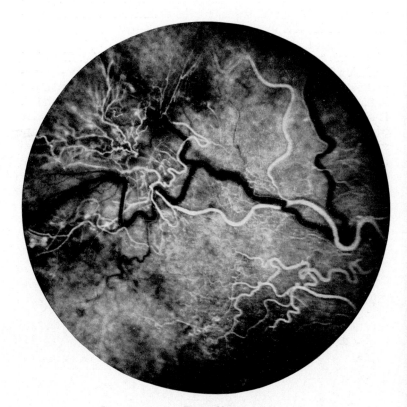

Figure 12

Clinical presentation: White woman aged 53 years.

Systemic features: Six years previously this patient had suffered a cerebral haemorrhage, a result of undiagnosed hypertension. A left-sided hemiplegia gradually recovered. Hypotensive therapy now maintains blood pressure in the region of 150/90.

Ocular symptoms: There had been sudden loss of vision in the right eye, perception of light only, returning over a 6-month period to 6/9. Initial examination revealed a right vitreous haemorrhage. As this cleared over a period of weeks many retinal changes were revealed.

Ophthalmoscopic findings: The region illustrated in *Plate 12*, the superior temporal area of the right eye, is typical of all quadrants of the right fundus. The retinal arteries are extremely tortuous, have a heightened surface reflex and are causing venous nipping at cross-over points. Highly refractile plaques in the arterial wall are visible half-way along its length. Towards the periphery, just beyond the view illustrated, the origin of the vitreous haemorrhage could be seen in a network of new retinal vessels.

Fluorescein angiogram: Arterial phase (*Figure 12*). The tortuosity of the retinal arteries is well depicted and the patency of the main artery, despite the atherosclerotic plaques in its wall, seems unimpaired. There is, however, gross narrowing of a branch arteriole at this site. The network of intra- and pre-retinal new vessels apparently arise from arterial vessels. They are seen towards the periphery and are presumed to be the result of local anoxia, secondary to arterial obstruction. The venous drainage is embarrassed as a result of the local overloading of the circulation from the extended arterial network. Venous engorgement and tortuosity are an expression of the imbalance in the retinal circulation.

13—Hypertension: Retinal Branch Vein Occlusion

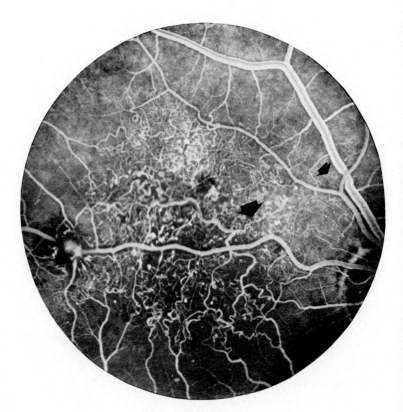

Figure 13

Clinical presentation: An active person with 8-year history of hypertension well controlled by drug therapy.

Systemic features: No clinical, cardiac or renal dysfunction.

Ocular symptoms: There had been sudden onset of blurred central vision in the right eye, 4 weeks prior to examination. The visual acuity was 6/24.

Ophthalmoscopic findings: A complete ring of lipid deposits (circinate retinopathy) surrounds the haemorrhagic lesion on the macular branch of the superior temporal retinal arteries (*Plate 13*). Some minor haemorrhages are scattered in this region which also shows mild retinal oedema. The location of the oedema and the lipid deposits account for the blurred central vision.

Fluorescein angiogram: Mid-venous phase (*Figure 13*). The haemorrhagic lesion of the macular branch of the superior temporal retinal artery is seen at the left of the picture. Between it and the optic disc on the right of the picture and the macula below, there is heavy capillary congestion and dilatation. The venous drainage of the area of retina supplied by the artery crossing the field is to the inferior temporal retinal vein below and the superior temporal retinal vein above. The tributary venules are clearly seen entering the superior main vein at right angles. To the right of the picture, where the superior temporal artery branches and crosses the vein, a branch venule has been obliterated. Its original course was from the site of indentation of the main vein, coursing down and laterally towards the artery. Its distal end and branches are still patent but terminate abruptly at the occluded venule (*arrowed*); this is the most significant feature of this angiogram. Because of this obstruction to the venous outflow, blood is diverted through other (collateral) channels which as a consequence of the extra blood flow become dilated. It can be seen from this angiogram that blood is diverted to venous outflow channels in all directions, that is, to the remaining patent branch vessels of the superior vein and also to the inferior vein. Microaneurysmal dilatations are evident at capillary levels.

This is a typical situation for exudation to occur, with gross vessel congestion. The late-phase angiogram showed widespread staining of the oedema fluid, including the macular area. Note in this angiogram that the dense lipid deposits seen in the colour photograph are not visible, that is, there is no recording of reflected blue light from the fundus. Only the presence of fluorescein is recorded and as lipid deposits do not imbibe the dye, they are invisible on a fluorescein angiogram.

14—Hypertension: *Arteriosclerosis*

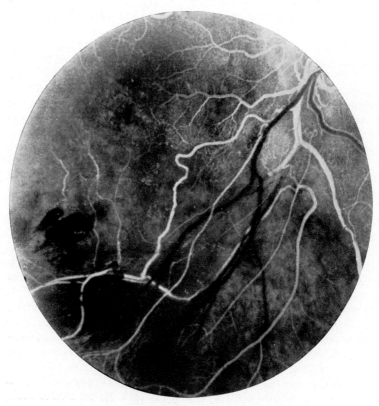

Figure 14 (a)

Clinical presentation: White man aged 48 years.

Systemic features: Recently discovered hypertension—190/110. Radiographic evidence of left ventricular enlargement. No albuminuria. The hypertension was discovered as a result of the patient's ocular symptoms.

Ocular symptoms: Loss of some vision in the right eye, visual acuity 6/24. Complete loss of the superior nasal and partial loss of the superior temporal visual field.

Ophthalmoscopic findings: Right eye. Apparent obliteration of the inferior temporal retinal artery with gross pipe-stem sheathing (*Plate 14*). The whitish-yellow occluded artery contrasts with the adjacent patent arteries which nevertheless show marked calibre variations. Lipid deposits and some small haemorrhages are scattered.

Fluorescein angiograms: A sequence of three angiograms to illustrate the basis of the retinopathy, the local response of the circulation to the new situation and finally the effect on the fundus of this pathology is presented in *Figures 14 (a), (b), (c).*

Arterial phase (a)

The inferior branch of the central retinal artery fills normally with dye at its origin, but there is an abrupt cessation of dye flow in the main temporal branch soon after its division into temporal and nasal branches. The non-fluorescent (black) remainder of the inferior temporal retinal artery and its branch are seen in the mid and lower aspects of the angiogram together with the noticeably non-fluorescent inferior temporal retinal vein. The inferior nasal retinal vein shows laminar fluorescence at this stage. A collateral channel is attempting to maintain arterial blood flow to the temporal side of the main artery; its tortuous route is well defined and its calibre variations are constant. Towards the nasal side (right) of the angiogram the narrow patent arterial channel maintains flow in the inferior branches of the inferior temporal artery.

Venous phase (b)

The inferior temporal vein is now fully fluorescent and arising from this venous side of the circulation, new retinal vessels are developing profusely, in the anoxic retina (*arrowed*). They are particularly seen below and temporal to the macula. This latter area is seen to be largely avascular, a few channels maintaining irregular contact with the superior retinal circulation. The occluded aspects of the inferior temporal artery remain non-fluorescent generally, although some wall staining with dye can be seen intermittently along its length. Black (haemorrhagic) areas are seen at the bottom left of the angiogram.

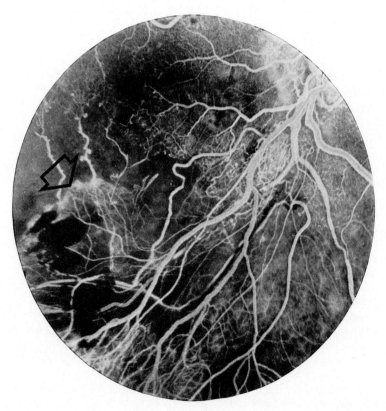

Figure 14 (b)

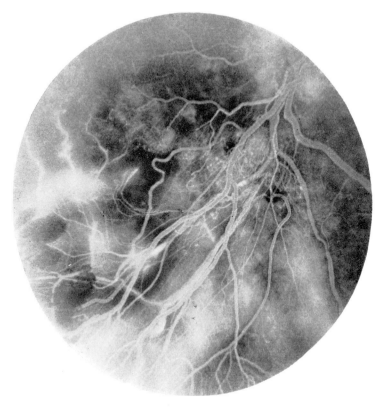

Figure 14 (c)

Late phase (c)

Three features are outstanding in this view:

(1) profuse leakage of dye has occurred from the areas of retinal neovascularization;

(2) retinal oedema is stained with varying intensity, throughout the field;

(3) damaged vessel walls are stained with fluorescein.

15—Malignant Hypertension

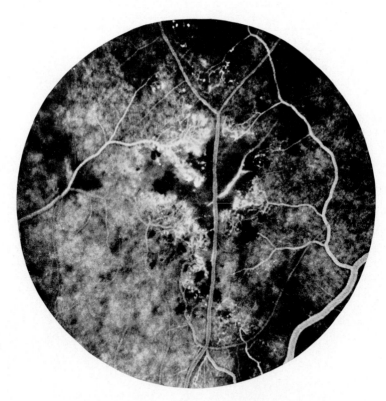

Figure 15

Clinical presentation: White man aged 32 years.

Systemic features: The patient was asymptomatic and presented complaining of his visual symptoms. On examination he was found to have a blood pressure of 200/140. There was no albuminuria.

Ocular symptoms: Blurring of vision in the right eye for 3 weeks, with some loss of the inferior field of vision on that side.

Ophthalmoscopic findings: The area illustrated above the right optic disc shows small vessel calibre irregularities and haemorrhages associated with an unusually straight retinal artery (*Plate 15*). Retinal soft exudates are seen on each side of the artery at the upper aspect of the photograph.

Fluorescein angiogram: From an informative series of angiograms, the one illustrated (*Figure 15*) was chosen from the retinal venous phase. It reveals the essential features of this retinopathy. The retinal artery bisecting the angiogram is unusually straightened in its course, and its branches, which are few in number, leave it almost at right angles. Although its fluorescence is fading, it is seen that its calibre is grossly irregular, similar to its branches. Many of them have been occluded at origin, although some branch stems can be seen emerging from the parent vessel. Endothelial damage and vessel necrosis constitute the underlying pathology. This is the response of these vessels to the hypertension and varying degrees of damage are seen. Some staining of the arterial wall has occurred, and there is gross staining of the vessel wall with dye leakage from a branch on the right, half-way up the picture. As a result of these arteriolar occlusions, the retina supplied by this artery is essentially avascular. The absent capillary circulation is denoted by darker areas adjacent to the artery some of which are occupied by the cotton wool patches which can be seen in the ophthalmoscopic view. Some are occupied haemorrhages, which appear as a contrasting black in the angiogram. Resulting from the cessation of blood flow, the venular side of the capillary bed has undergone generalized dilatation due to the anoxia of blood stagnation. Microaneurysm formation is also evident. Dye leakage from these vessels is profuse as a result of endothelial damage.

16—Malignant Hypertension

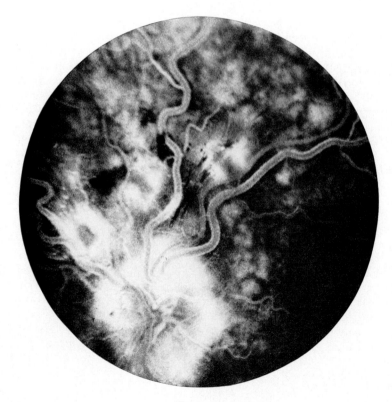

Figure 16

Clinical presentation: White woman aged 34 years.

Systemic features: Blood pressure 230/140. Abrupt onset of severe headaches and occasional nausea. Gross albuminuria.

Ocular symptoms: Abrupt onset of blurred vision with subsequent rapid deterioration.

Ophthalmoscopic findings: Tortuosity and irregular calibre of retinal arteries with congestion of all major retinal veins (*Plate 16*). Linear and flame-shaped haemorrhages radiate well beyond the optic disc region. Numerous cotton wool patches are illustrated in the field of view. Early papilloedema and diffuse retinal oedema add up to a *grade 4* hypertensive retinopathy.

Fluorescein angiogram: Later phase *Figure 16*. This phase is chosen to show the appearances of the optic disc in early papilloedema and the fluorescence of cotton wool patches. This develops as a result of dye-leakage from dilated capillaries surrounding the area of capillary closure which exist beneath retinal cotton wool patches. Fluorescein leaks from these dilated capillaries and microaneurysms which can also be seen, and diffuses into the cotton wool patch giving it a persistent, brilliant, fluffy fluorescence. In contrast, the retinal haemorrhages which are principally superficial, remain non-fluorescent. In early papilloedema, capillaries of the optic nerve head become incontinent to fluorescein, which diffuses well beyond the disc margin staining the oedema fluid. Finally, the congested and somewhat tortuous retinal veins can easily be identified by their residual fluorescence.

17—Malignant Hypertension

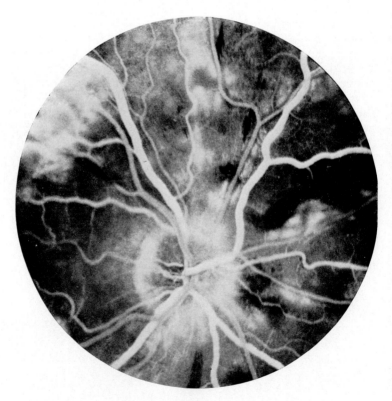

Figure 17

Clinical presentation: White woman aged 52 years.

Systemic features: Known hypertension for 5 years with renal damage and gross albuminuria. Serum albumin 1·6 g per 100 ml.

Ocular symptoms: Severe loss of vision in both eyes during the previous 3 months.

Ophthalmoscopic findings: From the regions of both optic discs, multiple linear retinal haemorrhages radiated in all directions (*Plate 17*). Intermingled with these were retinal cotton wool patches. In general there was diffuse fundus oedema.

Fluorescein angiogram: The principal feature is the staining of the retina with fluorescein, the result of dye leakage from retinal capillaries (*Figure 17*). Intermingled with staining areas are retinal haemorrhages which obscure some underlying detail. This angiogram in the retinal venous phase depicts a diffuse seepage of dye at the margins of the optic disc, that is, early papilloedema. Later phase angiograms showed widespread staining of the whole fundus with fluorescein.

The changes depicted here are essentially at the capillary level, and reflect the effects of the low serum albumin as much as the effects of high blood pressure.

18—Malignant Hypertension

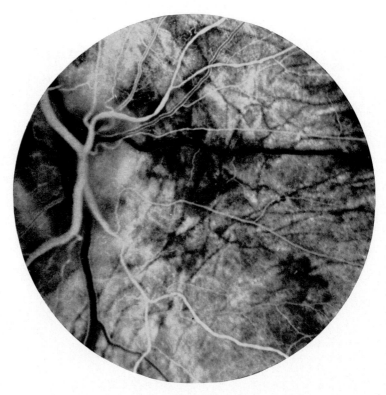

Figure 18

Clinical presentation: White man aged 47 years.

Systemic features: Four months previously, hypertension had been diagnosed after the patient had complained of feeling generally unwell, and more specifically of a headache and unusual thirst. He had gross albuminuria.

Ocular symptoms: At the time of diagnosis, the patient was suffering a rapid deterioration of vision in each eye. This proceeded until only perception of light remained.

Ophthalmoscopic findings: Ophthalmoscopy 4 months prior to the angiography revealed papilloedema with diffuse retinal oedema, widespread linear haemorrhages in the retina, cotton wool patches and gross arterial calibre irregularities. The patient's response to hypotensive therapy was good in the general sense, but his fundi never recovered to any satisfactory degree (*Plate 18*). The resultant picture in the right fundus is illustrated. There is secondary optic atrophy with pallor of the disc which had diffuse or woolly edges. The retinal arteries in view are very thin and irregular in calibre with retinal veins appearing interrupted where arteries cross.

Fluorescein angiogram: The angiogram (*Figure 18*) in the early venous phase demonstrates the aftermath of the severely raised blood pressure, the resultant papilloedema and fundus oedema. Attention is drawn to the network of black lines which occupy the background area of the angiogram. These represent folds in the retinal pigment epithelium, the result of oedema of the choroid, and its subsequent resolution. The elastic tissue in Bruch's membrane has been stretched and cannot return to its former dimension. Its wrinkling is evidenced by these folds in the overlying retinal pigment epithelium which are highlighted by fluorescence in the choroid. The calibre variations in the retinal arteries are the result of their exposure to extremely high blood pressures, destruction of the normal tissue of vessel walls and their replacement by fibrosis.

HYPERTENSION AND THE FUNDUS OF THE EYE

The maximum pressure exerted on the blood column in the systemic arterial system occurs during contraction of the left ventricle. This pressure is known as the systolic blood pressure and represents the response of the heart to the demand upon it created by the status of the peripheral resistance, that is, the tone of the arteriolar network throughout the body. A high systolic blood pressure results from a loss of flexibility in the arterioles.

The minimum pressure of blood in the arterial network is that found during relaxation of the left ventricle and is known as the diastolic blood pressure. Diastolic blood pressure is the minimum pressure that arterial vessels have to contain. A raised diastolic blood pressure therefore exerts a *continuous* effect on arteriole vessel walls and in that sense is a more serious effect than a raised systolic pressure.

The systemic effects of a persistently raised diastolic blood pressure on arterioles fall into 3 major groups.

(1) A reactive arteriolar sclerosis, that is found in vessels throughout the body.

(2) The development of microaneurysms on the perforating cerebral arteries.

(3) A fulminating effect—acute arteriolar fibrinoid necrosis.

Effects 1 and 3 are seen in the retinal circulation.

The response of the visible retinal blood vessels to hypertension is dependent on the initial state of these vessels. This in turn is dependent on the age of the patient and the state of ageing of the arterioles.

There is a gradual replacement of the muscle and elastic tissue of retinal arteriolar walls by fibrous tissue, an ageing process that results in narrower, paler, straighter vessels with more acute branchings. This situation is called involutionary sclerosis and is seen typically in patients aged over 60 years.

EFFECTS OF HYPERTENSION

On retinal vessels without ageing fibrosis

In the short term there may be no unusual findings.

With persistent hypertension a generalized constriction of retinal arterioles is the result of hypertonus. Straightening of these vessels and acute branching are features seen at this stage.

Persistent hypertonus gives way in time to permanent wall changes in the arterioles. An intermediate hyperplasia of connective tissue and elastic tissue is eventually replaced by fibrous tissue, that is, arteriolar sclerosis. The other effects of hypertension during this period and thereafter depend on the functional integrity of the retinal vessels. When this breaks down, local exudation and oedema occur, together with haemorrhages generally in the nerve fibre layer of the retina or subhyaloid in situation. Narrowing of arteriolar lumens or hyaline degeneration within the vessel walls, can cause arteriolar branch occlusions with obvious sequelae.

When arteries cross veins in the fundus, abnormalities occur which are characteristic features of hypertension.

Gunn's sign. -Apparent constriction of a vein by the artery crossing it.

Salus sign.—Displacement of the axis of a vein by an artery crossing it.

On retinal vessels with ageing fibrosis or involutionary sclerosis

Fibrosed segments of arterioles undergo passive dilatation and some tortuosity of the vessel is thus induced. Contractile segments, however, behave as above becoming hypertonic, narrowed, straight and pale and with acute very angled branches. In time the hypertonic segments undergo the series of changes already described above for the younger vessels. The state of any retinopathy thereafter depends on the functional integrity of the constituent vessels.

Malignant hypertension

The term refers to that group of hypertensive patients in whom the course of events is fulminating or rapidly progressive. Essentially, young arteries are destroyed by the persistent high pressure (diastolic usually between 140 and 160 mm Hg). Older arteries with a degree of ageing fibrosis in the arteriolar walls can withstand high pressures more successfully.

A differentiating feature of the retinopathy of malignant hypertension from the less severe forms of raised blood pressure is the consistent presence of optic disc oedema and diffuse retinal oedema —neuroretinopathy.

Studies in pathology have shown that arteriolar walls become thickened with swelling of cells and hyperplasia of elastic tissues. Focal arteriolar fibrinoid necrosis occurs, especially at arteriolar origins, and cotton wool patches result.

The general features of a malignant hypertensive retinopathy, arteriolar calibre variations, arteriolar occlusions, venous congestion and tortuosity, haemorrhages of various types, fundus oedema, lipid deposits, cotton wool patches and diffuse retinal oedema can be classified to give some idea of prognosis. According to Keith, Wagener and Barker (1939) 4 grades of malignant hypertensive retinopathy can usefully be described as follows.

(1) Slight constriction of vessels.

(2) Marked constriction of vessels with calibre variations; arterio-venous crossing phenomena.

(3) Superimposed on the above picture, haemorrhage and cotton wool patches.

(4) Additional: papilloedema, retinal oedema and gross lipid deposits (macular star).

19—Branch Retinal Artery Occlusion (Atherosclerosis)

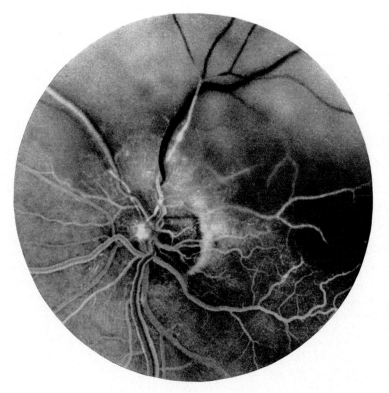

Figure 19

Clinical presentation: White man aged 65 years.

Systemic features: Angina pectoris and intermittent claudication.

Ocular features: Loss of the inferior field of vision of the left eye 12 hours previously.

Ophthalmoscopic findings: Retinal 'oedema' in the area of distribution of the upper branches of the central retinal artery, associated with severely attenuated retinal arteries (*Plate 19*).

Fluorescein angiogram: In contrast to the lower branches of the central retinal artery which fill normally with fluorescein, the upper aspect of this angiogram (*Figure 19*) shows no retinal circulation. The retinal arteries are severely attenuated and irregular, the calibres of the lumens of the superior branches of the central retinal artery are extremely narrowed at their origin from the central artery. A little fluorescein has permeated both of these vessels and demonstrates these features.

20—Central Retinal Artery Occlusion (Giant Cell Arteritis)

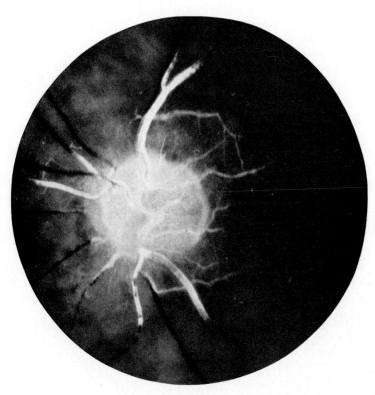

Figure 20 (a)

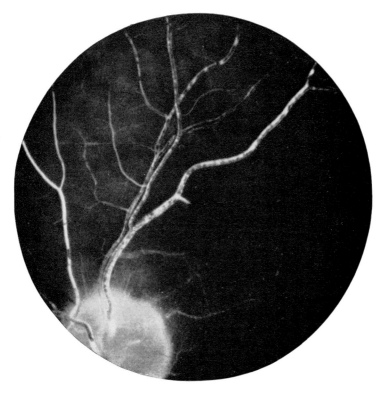

Figure 20 (b)

Clinical presentation: White man aged 67 years.

Systemic features: Six-months' history of headaches in the temporal regions. Palpation of the superficial temporal arteries revealed thickening and tenderness, and ESR (Westergren) was 84 mm in the first hour.

Ocular features: The patient suffered complete loss of vision in the left eye 24 hours previously.

Ophthalmoscopic findings: Left eye—generalized retinal 'oedema' contrasting with a 'cherry-red spot' at the macula, gross narrowing of the branches of the central retinal artery and 'cattle trucking' of the blood stream in the retinal veins (*Plate 20*).

Fluorescein angiogram: The central retinal artery and its branches fail to fill with fluorescein (*Figures 20a, b*). The brilliant fluorescence of the optic disc is the result of its blood supply from the choroid, that is, the optic disc is not supplied by the central retinal artery or its branches. Some of the fluorescein in the disc circulation is drained into tributaries of the central retinal vein and thus we see retrograde diffusion of fluorescein along the retinal veins. The cattle trucking effect in the venous branches is demonstrated as segments of blood alternate with the segments of fluorescent plasma.

Temporal arteritis

Destruction of the internal elastic layer with foreign body type giant-cell formation are the underlying histopathological changes in this disorder which manifests itself in several forms. Relevant to fundus disease is the affection of the temporal vessels which become thick-ened and tender and cause local headache. It is a disorder of the over 60s and ocular symptoms occur in about 40 per cent of cases. Ten to twenty per cent present with an occlusion of the central retinal artery or one of its major branches. Others present with visual loss and disc swelling—the result of optic nerve head ischaemia.

Diagnosis is suggested by the clinical findings, a markedly elevated sedimentation rate, and is confirmed by temporal artery biopsy. Treatment with systemic steroid preparations can reduce the inflammatory response and may preserve vision in the fellow eye.

The disc swelling and visual loss in the disorder is an ischaemic optic neuropathy which may be hard to differentiate, in less florid cases, from arteriosclerotic optic neuropathy.

Ischaemic optic neuropathy

Ischaemic optic neuropathy affects patients over 45 years of age, often in both eyes. The symptoms in both eyes may develop in a time-lapse of days to several years. The onset of the symptoms is sudden—loss of altitudinal visual field, mostly in the lower half, sometimes together with central vision deterioration. These patients always have some signs of generalized vascular disease (arterio-sclerosis, hypertension). When temporal artery biopsy is done, specimens usually show arteriosclerotic arterial changes, but never arteritis.

The ophthalmoscopic picture is of a pale papilloedema with some spindle-shaped haemorrhages around the disc. The disc of the other eye can be pale with sharp margins, resembling the picture of Foster Kennedy syndrome (*see* page 55). The disc swelling disappears quite quickly, leaving an optic atrophy with slightly blurred disc margins and sheathing of the central artery branches on the disc.

There is no specific therapy although steroids are frequently given. There may be some degree of spontaneous remission.

21—Diabetes Mellitus

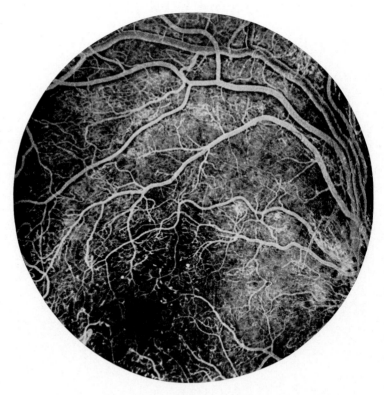

Figure 21

Clinical presentation: White woman aged 23 years.

Systemic features: Sixteen-year history of diabetes; insulin—80 units daily.

Ocular features: This patient was virtually blind in her left eye, but had normal sight in her right eye.

Ophthalmoscopic features: The left eye showed an almost total retinal detachment secondary to advanced retinitis proliferans. Right eye; apart from scattered microaneurysms and dot haemorrhages, the fundus in this eye appeared substantially normal (*Plate 21*).

Fluorescein angiogram: (Right) In contrast to the normal appearances by ophthalmoscopy, the angiogram reveals generalized and extensive capillary dilatation (*Figure 21*). In the foveal area, a few micro-aneurysms are seen, and the perifoveal capillary arcades are some-what distorted as well as dilated. Superimposed on this picture is evidence of generalized intraretinal new vessel formation. The major retinal arteries and veins appear angiographically normal. The later phase photographs reveal extensive intraretinal staining with fluores-cein, the result of leakage of dye from the extensive network of de-veloping new vessels.

22—Diabetes Mellitus

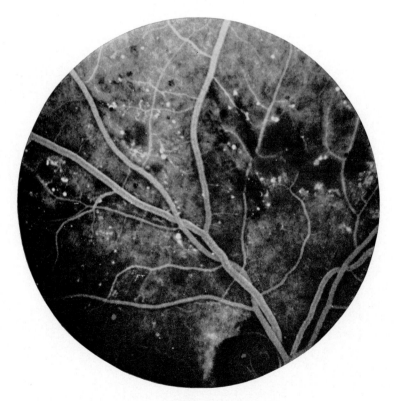

Figure 22

Clinical presentation: White man aged 32 years.

Systemic features: Patient was a known diabetic for 10 years, on 32 units of insulin daily. He was a completely fit patient and had no albuminuria.

Ocular features: Patient had no eye symptoms. His diabetic retinopathy was discovered as a result of routine examination.

Ophthalmoscopic findings: Microaneurysms were abundant in both fundi. A selective area above the right optic disc, illustrated in *Plate 22*, showed multiple coalescent retinal exudates with associated dot and linear haemorrhages.

Fluorescein angiogram: Far more microaneurysms were demonstrated by angiography (*Figure 22*) than could be noted ophthalmoscopically. The linear haemorrhages in the retinal nerve fibre layer, contrast black against the fluorescent background. The areas of exudation in the retina, are seen to be areas of non-perfusion of the capillary bed, contrasting with the surrounding areas. The retinal arteries and veins were of normal calibre and showed no unusual angiographic features.

Zones of capillary closure, microaneurysm formation and minor retinal haemorrhages are some of the earliest features of diabetic retinopathy.

23—Diabetes Mellitus

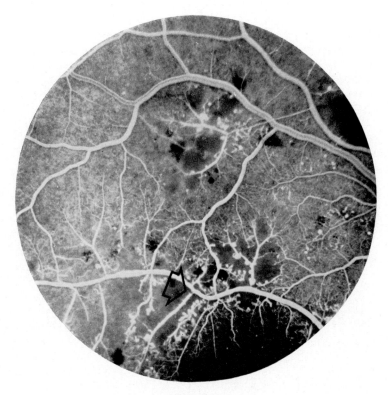

Figure 23

Clinical presentation: White man aged 54 years.

Systemic features: Patient was a known diabetic for 10 years, on 55 units of insulin daily. He had experienced 2 episodes of myocardial infarction in the past 18 months. His right leg had been amputated following vascular insufficiency and gangrene.

Ocular symptoms: Blurring of vision in both eyes, and blind spots in the fields of vision.

Ophthalmoscopic findings: The major features of this retinopathy were the retinal soft exudates. About 15 large soft exudates were located in the central areas of each fundus. The superior temporal vessel area of the right fundus, illustrated in *Plate 23*, shows several soft exudates with associated microaneurysms and retinal haemorrhages. A large retinal hard exudate is seen just above the superior temporal artery.

Fluorescein angiogram: The clear definition of the retinal capillary bed in general (*Figure 23*) contrasts with several areas of capillary closure (or non-perfusion). Each of these areas additionally shows dilatation of the surrounding capillaries, multiple microaneurysm formation on vessels in the region, and arteriole branch occlusions. One arteriole in particular (*arrowed*) has its own lumen almost occluded at its origin, and branches stemming from it have all been occluded almost at source. In contrast to the fluorescent microaneurysms the scattered retinal haemorrhages appear black (non-fluorescent). Although the retinal veins are normal in calibre, the large retinal artery crossing the picture shows calibre variation and later angiograms revealed persistent staining of its wall indicating a severe degree of endothelium and wall damage.

The occlusive arteriopathy which is the key feature of this patient's retinopathy is well reflected in his systemic features with vascular occlusive episodes in his coronary arteries, limb arteries and renal arteries.

24—Diabetes Mellitus and Hypertension

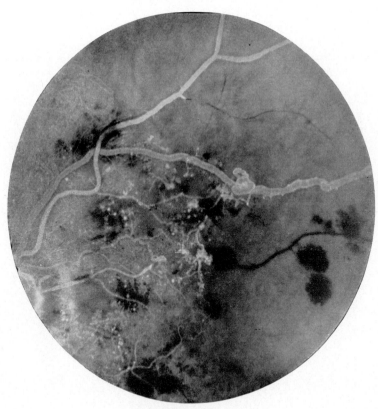

Figure 24

Clinical presentation: White man aged 64 years.

Systemic features: Fifteen-year history of diabetes controlled by oral therapy and diet. Seven years' history elevated blood pressure maintained by hypotensive therapy at 160/100 level.

Ocular symptoms: Deterioration of vision over a 5-year period. Visual acuity, right eye 6/18; left eye 6/60.

Ophthalmoscopic findings: Left eye. The region illustrated in *Plate 24* is lateral to the optic disc. The superior temporal retinal vein crosses the photograph, part of the superior temporal artery is seen above it. Branches of the superior temporal artery cannot be seen clearly. One branch is markedly arteriosclerotic.

The superior temporal retinal vein runs an irregular course. It shows a complete loop in the centre of the picture and thereafter it is somewhat dilated. Several patches of lipid deposits occupy the upper aspects of the area whereas several patches of intraretinal haemorrhage are seen in the lower aspect. Microaneurysms are plentiful.

Fluorescein angiogram: The superior temporal retinal artery is seen in its entirety from the optic disc below to its first major division above (*Figure 24*). Its branch arterioles emanating at 90 degrees are largely occluded at source; their origins can just be seen. These non-fluorescent vessels can be seen as black threads against the diffuse background fluorescence from the choroid. The venous irregularities can be worked out in detail from this view. The retinal capillary circulation has largely disappeared leaving a view of choroidal fluorescence through a generally oedematous retina.

25—Diabetes Mellitus

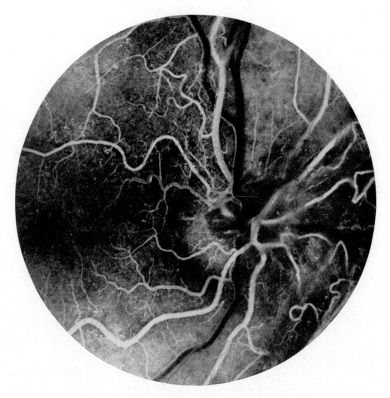

Figure 25

Clinical presentation: White man aged 37 years.

Systemic features: Patient was a known diabetic for 20 years on 65 units of insulin daily. He was a fit person but had albuminuria.

Ocular symptoms: Three years before there had been loss of vision in the left eye; he was now complaining of deteriorating vision in the right eye.

Ophthalmoscopic findings: The left eye was blind, the result of retinitis proliferans and recurrent vitreous haemorrhage. The right eye, illustrated in *Plate 25*, shows advancing retinitis proliferans with filmy fibrous tissue, and fine-calibre blood vessels pushing forwards from the region of the optic disc into the vitreous of the eye. Retinal traction effects of the fibrous tissue can be seen temporal to the optic disc with fine retinal folds or stress lines emanating from the point of traction above the optic disc. Retinal details on the nasal side of the optic disc are obscured by the overlying retinitis proliferans.

Fluorescein angiogram: In this early phase picture (*Figure 25*) immediate seepage of dye from the proliferating vessels on the nasal side of the optic disc casts a hazy fluorescent veil over the fundus features. Some tortuous arterial vessels can be seen amidst the fibrous tissues. (In later phase, the fluorescence from these areas was massive.) On the temporal side of the disc, generalized capillary dilatation, microaneurysms and intraretinal new vessels are all demonstrated, more clearly so in the superior temporal region.

26—Diabetes Mellitus

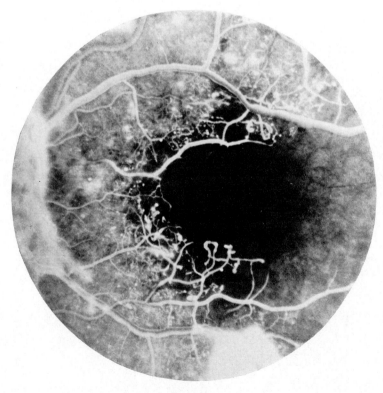

Figure 26

Clinical presentation: White man aged 26 years.

Systemic features: Patient had been diabetic for 21 years maintained on daily insulin of 60 units and diet.

Ocular symptoms: Right eye, visual acuity 6/18. There had been gradual deterioration of vision due to retinitis proliferans with obscuration of the macula by new retinal vessels. Left eye, visual acuity 6/60. This eye had had poor central vision for 2 years, the peripheral field of vision remained intact.

Ophthalmoscopic findings: Left eye, a lacework of new retinal vessels runs superficial to the optic disc and along the major vessels (*Plate 26*). There is evidence of intraretinal new vessel formation. Micro-aneurysms and small haemorrhages abound. There is general retinal oedema.

Fluorescein angiogram: The venous phase is illustrated in *Figure 26*. Dye leakage and tissue staining in the region of the optic disc from superficial neovascularization is seen at the left aspect of the picture. The macular area, centrally, is strikingly avascular. Its pigmentation obscures the deeper choroidal fluorescence and, therefore, highlights the remaining retinal circulation in its region. The macular branch of the superior temporal artery is patent initially, but is occluded just temporal to the macula. Its wall is vividly stained with dye. The branch arterioles are occluded at source, some stems can just be seen. The avascular retina centrally contrasts with the retinal vessel dilatation elsewhere and new vessel formation at various stages of development. Budding new vessels from a branch venule are well defined below. The vascularized retina is heavily stained with fluorescein indicating its degree of oedema.

27—Diabetes Mellitus

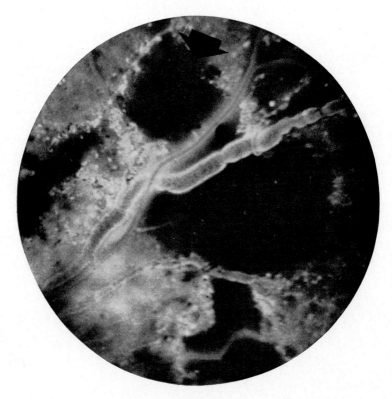

Figure 27

Clinical presentation: White woman aged 24 years.

Systemic features: Patient had been diabetic for 17 years, requiring a daily maintenance dose of 60 units of insulin. She had mild albuminuria.

Ocular symptoms: There was a 3-year history of noting increasing numbers of blind spots in both fields of vision. Symptoms had been exacerbated during recent pregnancy.

Ophthalmoscopic findings: Both fundi showed widespread venous engorgement with tortuosity of veins, repeated venous nipping giving sausage-like segments (*Plate 27*). Various types of retinal haemorrhages were scattered throughout both fundi, including dot and blob haemorrhages and small subhyaloid haemorrhages. Soft and hard retinal exudates were numerous at the posterior poles of both eyes and new retinal vessels were seen especially in the regions of the optic discs.

Fluorescein angiogram: A portion of the upper temporal region of the left fundus is illustrated in *Figure 27*. This photograph was taken $1\frac{1}{2}$ minutes after injection of dye. Thus the intravascular concentration of dye has already fallen sharply after the initial dye transit. Comparison with the colour photograph reveals that large areas of this fundus, contain non-functioning retinal capillaries. These areas of capillary closure (*arrowed*), are generally surrounded by dilated capillaries some of which bear microaneurysms. The retinal capillaries elsewhere in the field of view are incontinent to fluorescein which consequently has stained those regions of the fundus. The microaneurysms show persistent fluorescence, and contrast with the non-fluorescent dot and blob haemorrhages scattered throughout the field. The distension and segmentation of the superior temporal vein is dramatic, its wall staining with fluorescein is a result of the relative stagnation of blood flow, anoxia and consequent endothelial damage.

DIABETIC RETINOPATHY

Diabetes is the most important systemic cause of blindness in Great Britain—approximately 7 per cent (700 cases) of new blind registrations each year, a figure likely to rise as life expectancy increases with improved anti-diabetic therapy, coupled with our inability to prevent retinal complications.

Photographic studies of the human diabetic retina *in vivo* are now

97

adding significantly to our knowledge of this condition, by enabling a detailed recording of the natural history of the angiopathy to be made and by the recording of the detailed response to treatment. The most important lesions of the retinopathy are to be found in channels not visible by ophthalmoscopy or by colour photography, that is, in the capillaries. Contrast angiography not only demonstrates capillaries but additionally reveals their abnormal function in terms of altered dye flow patterns, dye leakage and vessel wall staining.

Based on fluorescein angiographic appearances the earliest lesions in the retinopathy are found in the capillary bed and include microaneurysms, generalized capillary dilatation and areas of capillary closure. Microaneurysms most commonly saccular in type, are always associated with non-perfused capillaries. In the earliest cases they have a focal distribution but as the condition becomes more severe they become generally distributed over the posterior pole. They appear as fluorescent dots of less than 30 μm diameter. Larger ones are commonly seen associated with cotton wool spots. Confusion of microaneurysms with other fluorescent spots, for example those due to drusen or capillary loops, can be resolved by studying the angiographic sequence. Not all microaneurysms perfuse with fluorescein and thus may be confused with dot haemorrhages.

The generalized dilatation of retinal capillaries, which is a feature of advancing retinopathy, allows easier demonstration of these channels by angiography compared with the normal. Capillary closure, the earliest sign of diabetic retinopathy according to some workers, is indicated by black (non-perfused) areas interrupting the capillary pattern. Areas of capillary closure vary from 1 to several millimetres square. The absence of capillary perfusion in relation to retinal soft exudates is well recognized, dilated channels around soft exudates can usually be seen, dye flow through them is slow and they generally leak dye. In more severe retinopathies, occluded branch arterioles give rise to large areas of non-perfused capillaries. Arteriovenous communications across areas of capillary closure are often mistakenly termed shunt vessels, for their presence may follow longstanding capillary closure. Late revascularization of non-perfused capillaries in small areas has been seen.

Following in the wake of small vessel abnormalities, large vessel changes occur and are graphically demonstrated by fluorescein angiography. These include arterial lumen calibre variations, focal narrowing of branch arterioles at their origins, with distal dilatations; dilatation, tortuosity and looping of retinal veins with a marked tendency towards wall staining with fluorescein, emphasizing these appearances.

New retinal vessels are either intraretinal or preretinal. Intra-retinal new vessels appear as dilated channels on the venous side of the circulation; they do not always leak dye in early phase contrasting with preretinal vessels which are completely incontinent to fluores-cein. New vessels on the optic disc may at least in part arise from the ciliary-choroidal circulation according to angiographic evidence.

28—Iron Deficiency Anaemia
(Haemoglobin 25 per cent)

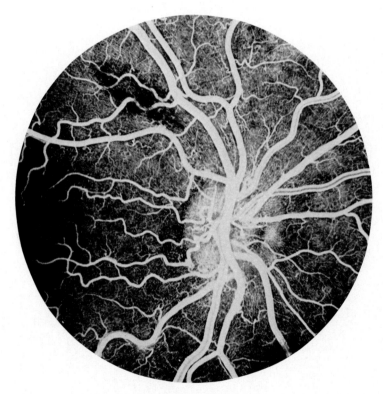

Figure 28

Clinical presentation: White woman aged 19 years.

Systemic features: General weakness and pallor of gradual onset over a six-month period. Menorrhagia for 3 years.

Ocular symptoms: The patient complained of blurring of vision in both eyes and noted blind spots in her field of vision.

Ophthalmoscopic findings: Both fundi showed unusual pallor. Linear and flame-shaped haemorrhages were scattered over both retinas. The right fundus, illustrated in *Plate 28*, shows the general pallor, but the optic disc is quite pink in colour. Between the superior temporal artery and vein, linear haemorrhages are seen, indicating superficial intraretinal bleeding (in the nerve fibre layer).

Fluorescein angiogram: The superb definition (*Figure 28*) of the vessels of the retinal circulation including the capillaries is a direct result of the degree of anaemia. The absorption spectrum of haemoglobin overlaps the emission spectrum of a blood fluorescein–fluorescent mixture. Consequently there is less absorption of emitted fluorescence in the severely anaemic patient, hence the unmasking of all the details seen in this field. The intraretinal haemorrhages do not absorb fluorescein and, therefore, appear a non-fluorescent black.

Additionally, as the circulation time is decreased in an anaemic patient even at rest, the passage of dye through the retinal circulation is extremely rapid. Re-circulation occurred in this patient within 12 seconds (normal range 23–35 seconds).

Additional notes: Fundus changes appear only if the haemoglobin is less than 50 per cent usually only below 35 per cent. The colour of the whole fundus is pale, an effect less marked than skin pallor.

The arteries are widened and the artery/vein ratio tends toward 1:1. The colour of arteries is brighter and their walls are more translucent. Flame-shaped (nerve layer) haemorrhages and cotton wool patches may feature rarely. Most changes are reversible, no scars remain and vision should be unaffected with successful treatment of the anaemia.

Pathogenesis: It is suspected that capillary endothelium damage results from a low intravascular oxygen tension.

29—Sickle-cell Anaemia

Clinical presentation: Negro (West Indian) woman aged 32 years.

Systemic features: This patient was asymptomatic apart from her eye complaint. Laboratory investigation revealed characteristic sickling of the red cells, electrophoretic studies demonstrated abnormal haemoglobin with predominant C haemoglobin.

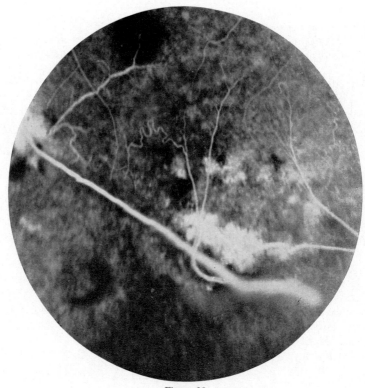

Figure 29

Ocular symptoms: Sudden loss of vision in the left eye to perception of light only, recovered over a period of 4 months during which time there was spontaneous clearing of a vitreous haemorrhage.

Ophthalmoscopic findings: Ophthalmoscopy then revealed peripheral retinal changes including tortuosity of retinal veins, associated haemorrhages and microaneurysms. In one area, neovascularization was marked and fibrosis within the vitreous was causing traction effects on these and normal retinal vessels. Such an area is illustrated in *Plate 29*. In the foreground of the picture, in focus, is a fibrotic band within the vitreous which is ensheathing and pulling the retinal vein from its retinal location into the vitreous cavity.

Fluorescein angiogram: The retinal background to the local site of vitreous traction is shown in *Figure 29*. The retinal vein is being pulled into the vitreous, becoming out of focus as it comes forward. In the background, retinal haemorrhages appear black and the neo-vascularization is identified by zones of fluorescent staining, the result of leakage from the new vessels. New retinal vessels at these sites typically take a fan-shaped configuration.

The clinical course of this eye was typical of many of such patients. Recurrent vitreous haemorrhage results in further intravitreal fibro-sis and retinal traction detachment. Blindness is the end result. These features make this a condition which is exceedingly difficult to treat.

Additional notes: Sickle-cell anaemia belongs to the haemoglobino-pathies of the S and C type.

The main feature of this disease is the sickling of the red blood cells in lower oxygen concentration, because of the insolubility of the reduced haemoglobin.

In the retina the changes are in the peripheral vessels due to is-chaemia and thrombosis. The changes are in stages as follows.

(1) Fullness and tortuosity of the veins.

(2) Additional neovascularization and telangiectasia with micro-aneurysm formation.

(3) Choroidoretinal degeneration with capillary thrombosis, microaneurysms and retinal haemorrhages.

(4) Retinitis proliferans, recurrent vitreous haemorrhages, intra-vitreal fibrosis with retinal traction detachment.

Other less common changes are angioid streaks and central retinal artery occlusion.

This retinopathy occurs in the S–C haemoglobinopathy, while in the S–S type only changes of grade 1 occur.

Sickle-cell disease occurs in homozygous patients while sickle-cell trait occurs in the heterozygotes who do not develop retinal changes.

30—Pernicious Anaemia

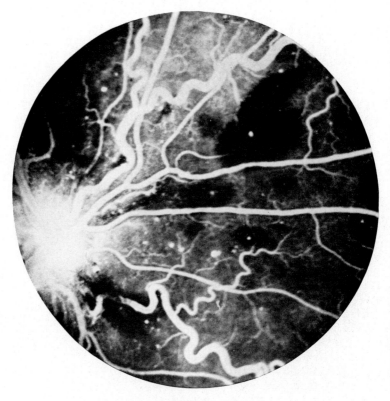

Figure 30

Clinical presentation: White woman aged 37 years.

Systemic features: Dyspnoea, ankle oedema, weight loss, anorexia, vomiting and passing blood per rectum. The patient's hair was completely white and very dry, she looked 70 years of age. Haemoglobin 22 per cent; white cells 4,900 per mm^3; platelets 39,000 per mm^3; MCV 107.

Ocular symptoms: Severe loss of vision in both eyes for at least one month, visual acuity less than 6/60 each eye.

Ophthalmoscopic findings: Right eye; linear, spindle-shaped, flame-shaped and confluent haemorrhages, principally in the nerve fibre layer, are scattered all around the optic disc and extend to the equator of the eye (*Plate 30*). The larger haemorrhages surround a central pale spot. The retinal veins are congested and very tortuous in their course.

Fluorescein angiogram: Venous phase (*Figure 30*). Widening and tortuosity of the retinal veins is accompanied by dilatation of the retinal arteries. Capillary congestion near and on the optic disc has already resulted in dye leakage which continued through into late phase, when widespread retinal staining with dye occurred around the disc.

The haemorrhages are non-fluorescent but each haemorrhage contains at least one large aneurysm which tends to be central and corresponds to the pale zone in the colour photograph. Many more microaneurysms are seen.

Additional notes: The retinopathy is the result of tissue hypoxia. Its general similarity to the hyperviscosity syndrome retinopathy is interesting for circulatory *stasis* in that condition also results in tissue hypoxia.

The typical findings in this disease are haemorrhages with white centres, but less outstanding than in leukaemia. The haemorrhages are round or flame-shaped, and blood vessels are wider but lack the typical colour contrast between arteries and veins, as in other types of anaemia.

31—Waldenström's Macroglobulinaemia

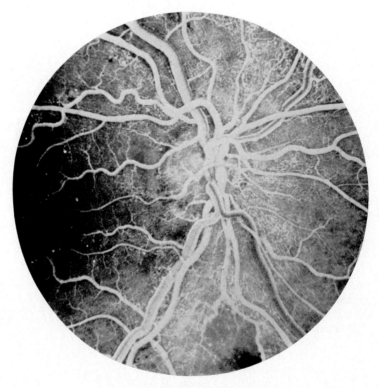

Figure 31

Clinical presentation: White man aged 55 years.

Systemic features: Six-month history of recurrent pyrexia, fatigue, dizziness, dyspnoea on exertion, and a bleeding tendency from nose, gums and haemorrhoids. Serum proteins: albumin 2·9 g/100 ml, globulin 7·5 g/100 ml (gammaglobulin 4·7 g/100 ml).

Ocular symptoms: Recent deterioration in vision, 6/18 in each eye.

Ophthalmoscopic findings: The most striking feature of the patient's fundi were the dark, engorged, irregularly dilated veins and widespread blob-type haemorrhages (*Plate 31a*). The arteries were regular in appearance, many blob and flame-shaped haemorrhages were evident, mainly between disc and macula. The area illustrated below the right optic disc, shows a soft retinal exudate and the characteristic 'string of sausages' appearance of the retinal veins. The left fundus shows more gross venous engorgement (*Plate 31b*).

Fluorescein angiogram: The circumpapillary net of retinal capillaries is clearly seen and shows generalized axial dilatation and some tortuosity (*Figure 31*). Fusiform and saccular aneurysmal dilatations are visible in all quadrants. A few linear and some dot haemorrhages are scattered throughout the field. An area of capillary closure in relation to the retinal soft exudates, visible in the colour illustration, is seen below the optic disc in the lowest part of the field. Retinal vein engorgement is well shown.

The interval between injection of dye and its arrival in the retinal circulation was unusually long in this patient—over 30 seconds (normal 10 seconds) and the retinal circulation time was extremely slow.

Additional notes: Waldenström's macroglobulinaemia is one of the hyperviscosity syndromes where thickening of the blood results in slowing of the circulation and stagnation, with resultant local anoxia. The retinal changes reflect this general situation and the response to slowing of the circulation is one of increasing congestion with resultant capillary dilatation, aneurysm formation and retinal haemorrhage. The retinopathy can be reversed by plasmaphaeresis which decreases serum protein concentration and, therefore, the hyperviscosity.

Other hyperviscosity syndromes include myelomatosis, cryoglobulinaemia and polycythaemia. Essentially, the retinopathies of the hyperviscosity syndromes contain the above features in greater or lesser degree.

32—Behçet's Disease

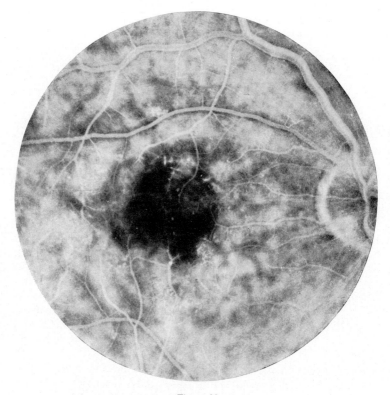

Figure 32

Clinical presentation: White man aged 32 years.

Systemic features: Five-year history of oral and genital ulceration.

Ocular features: Three-year history of recurrent anterior uveitis. The patient complained of recent further deterioration of vision in each eye.

Ophthalmoscopic findings: Both fundi showed oedema of the posterior poles most marked in the macular regions (*Plate 32*). Particular features which could be differentiated, included scattered retinal haemorrhages and some dot-like exudates.

Fluorescein angiogram: Evidence of retinal vasculitis is shown in *Figure 32*. The retinal capillaries in the field of view are generally permeable to fluorescein which, leaking out of the vessel walls, stains the surrounding retina, giving the whole of the posterior pole a diffuse but brilliant fluorescence. Particular features in the retinal vessels are the involvement of retinal arteries, capillaries and veins. However, it is generally at the capillary level that most signs are seen. Many capillaries are occluded whereas others are dilated and microaneurysm formation is abundant. Terminal arterioles in the macular region are occluded and the vessel walls are stained with dye in contrast to the non-fluorescent fundus around these vessels resulting from lack of dye transport.

It is these affections of the retinal vessels that result in the ophthalmoscopic appearance of diffuse retinal oedema. The staining of the oedema fluid and the abnormal vessels by fluorescein identifies the area of pathology.

Additional notes: The majority of patients with Behçet's disease who have eye involvement suffer a severe form of anterior uveitis. Posterior segment disease affects only a minority. Ophthalmoscopic features include diffusely scattered exudates in the retina, flame-shaped and preretinal haemorrhages. Vitreous haemorrhage may induce vascular proliferation.

Individual retinal blood vessels show calibre variations and sheathing by cellular infiltration. There are features of periarteritis and periphlebitis. Attendant macular oedema interferes with central vision. Resolution of the acute phase of the retinopathy can be followed by pigmentary changes in the fundus.

33—*Polyarteritis Nodosa*

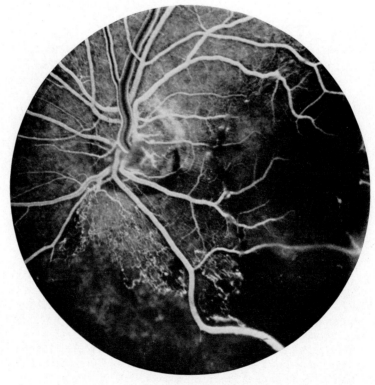

Figure 33 (*a*)

Clinical presentation: Indian man aged 25 years.

Systemic features: Presented as an acute illness with nausea, vomiting and anorexia. On examination he was found to have albuminuria, haematuria and he was hypertensive. The course of events was rapid and this patient died within 4 weeks of onset of symptoms. Midway through this period he suffered acute loss of vision in his left eye.

Ophthalmoscopic findings: Widespread retinal haemorrhages were the striking feature of this retinopathy. They were located principally in the macular region where subhyaloid and deeper haemorrhages obscured much of the retina. Examination of the region of the optic disc illustrated in *Plate 33*, showed that the inferior temporal retinal vein was completely obliterated.

Fluorescein angiogram: The macular region was largely obscured by haemorrhage. In the region of the optic disc (*Figure 33a*), the circulatory changes demonstrated include an absence of the inferior retinal circulation. Here, dilated radial circumpapillary capillaries, some with microaneurysmal dilatations were attempting to compensate for the vein occlusion. In contrast, the superior retinal vein was rather engorged as it coped with some extra venous drainage. The second angiogram of peripheral retina (*Figure 33b*) shows the widespread effects of the arteritis in later phase. The normal competence of the arterial walls has disappeared as a result of inflammation (arteritis) and periarterial diffusion of the fluorescein is very evident.

Additional notes: This disease belongs to the group of the collagen disorders. The fundus changes are very typical and have a value in the clinical diagnosis but they appear only in 20 per cent of cases. The disease usually affects adult men (20–40 years of age). The life expectancy is very poor, only 5–6 months

The fundus changes resemble those of 'albuminuric retinitis'. The vessels show calibre variations, haemorrhages and exudates abound.

Intraretinal and subretinal exudates give the picture of disseminated choroiditis. Bilateral serous retinal detachment, central artery or vein occlusion, and papilloedema also feature. The histological features

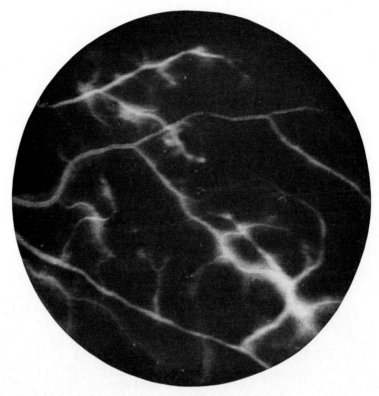

Figure 33 (b)

show 4 stages (according to Arkin): (1) degenerative; (2) inflammatory; (3) formation of granulation tissue; (4) healing stage—obliteration of the vessel lumen. These changes appear mainly in the
choroidal vessels.

34—*Wegener's Granulomatosis*

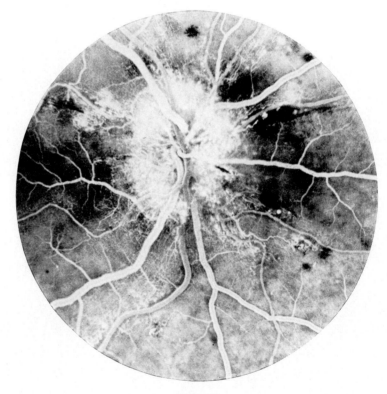

Figure 34

Clinical presentation: White man aged 42 years.

Systemic features: Severe hypertension.

Ocular features: Three-month history of blurred vision in each eye.

Ophthalmoscopic findings: The right optic disc region is illustrated in *Plate 34*. Diffuse swelling of the optic disc with loss of the central physiological cup. The optic disc oedema is continuous with the diffuse retinal oedema. Linear retinal haemorrhages radiate around the optic disc and are interspersed with punctate hard retinal exudates.

Fluorescein angiogram: Retinal venous phase. The gross dilatation of the capillaries on the optic nerve head extends irregularly into all quadrants of the retina with dilatation of the radial retinal capillaries (*Figure 34*). The capillaries on the disc are already leaking fluorescein which is staining the oedema of the optic nerve head and early leakage can be seen from the radial retinal capillaries in all fields. Microaneurysmal dilatations are numerous. The linear retinal haemorrhages are non-fluorescent and contrast against the background.

These appearances are suggestive of a central retinal vasculitis with inflammatory infiltration of the central retinal vessels, reflected in the angiographic view by the capillary congestive changes and resultant retinal oedema.

Additional notes: This disease is a variant of polyarteritis nodosa. Here the affected vessels are also small arteries and arterioles together with upper respiratory tract granulomas. Ocular changes appear only in a small percentage of patients. Lesions are most common in the choroid causing cotton wool exudates principally in the retina around the optic disc. The retinal vessels may be normal or show hypertensive changes. Severe involvement of the choroid may lead to subretinal oedema and serous detachment.

In the healing stage, patches of atrophy develop in the choroid and retinal pigment epithelium.

35—Eales' Disease

Clinical presentation: White man aged 38 years.

Systemic features: A fit man with no general symptoms or abnormal clinical findings.

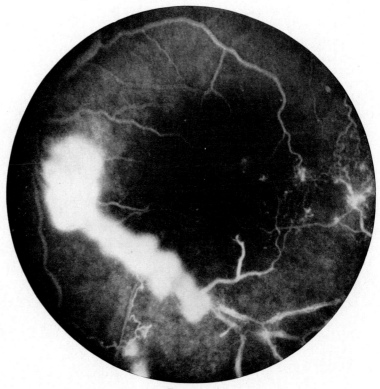

Figure 35

Ocular symptoms: Presented with sudden loss of vision in the left eye 2 years ago. The patient was found to have a complete vitreous haemorrhage in that eye. When this had cleared some 4 months later, evidence of Eales' disease, retinal periphlebitis, was found. Peripheral retinal neovascularization was treated by photocoagulation. He again succumbed to a vitreous haemorrhage and it took 6 months to clear.

Ophthalmoscopic findings: Left eye. Gross sheathing of the inferior temporal retinal vein and a frond of new vessels arise near the optic disc and run forwards through the vitreous to almost touch the back of the crystalline lens (*Plate 35*). As the retinal camera has a shallow depth of field, this illustration has concentrated on the frond of new vessels. In the background, out of focus, the optic disc can be seen to the left and the macula to the right. The situation has been reversed in the accompanying fluorescein angiogram so that the fundus is in sharp focus and the new vessels are out of focus in the foreground.

Fluorescein angiogram: Later phase. Dye leakage from the new vessels obscures their intrinsic pattern but identifies their location (*Figure 35*). They arise from the inferior temporal retinal vein which is grossly abnormal. Although it is largely obscured in this view, some of its branches can be seen below. They do contain dye, but the vessel walls are heavily stained with dye which is also leaking into the adjacent tissues.

A diversion of the circulation lateral to the macula is seen and represents an attempt to return some blood through the superior retinal venous network.

Close inspection of the branches of the inferior retinal vein reveals the presence of intramural new retinal vessels.

Additional notes: This disease occurs mainly in men 20–40 years of age. It is a disease of the peripheral retinal veins causing recurrent haemorrhages.

The small peripheral veins show white sheathing of the wall with small retinal haemorrhages around them. If the haemorrhages are large they may break through the hyaloid membrane and cause visual disturbances. These vitreous haemorrhages absorb spontaneously, but have a tendency to recur. After several haemorrhages there is connective tissue growth—retinitis proliferans—with new vessel formation into the vitreous and secondary retinal detachment. The cause of the disease is unknown but tuberculosis was thought to be the main cause and, therefore, antispecific therapy was common.

The more modern therapy is photocoagulation of the small veins, but it is successful only in the earlier stages.

36—Miliary Tuberculosis

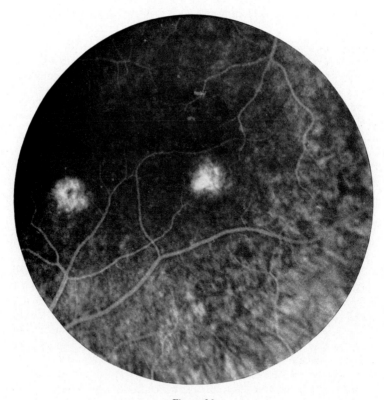

Figure 36

Clinical presentation: White man aged 28 years.

Systemic features: Acute miliary tuberculosis, principally affecting the lungs.

Ocular features: The patient was asymptomatic from the ocular point of view but ophthalmoscopy revealed the presence of choroidal tubercles.

Ophthalmoscopic findings: The miliary choroidal tubercles appeared as whitish raised foci of inflammation, about one-third of a disc diameter across (*Plate 36*). Each fundus showed 8 such lesions scattered around the posterior poles.

Fluorescein angiogram: Later phase. The miliary tubercles have stained with fluorescein and contrast against the darker background, the fading choroidal fluorescence (*Figure 36*). Foci of inflammation stain early with fluorescein which identifies their state of activity.

Additional notes: In the acute miliary form of tuberculosis, the bacteria reach the choroid through the posterior ciliary arteries, hence the localization of the lesions at the posterior pole. The white-grey foci of inflammation vary in size from pinpoint to a disc diameter. When they disappear there may be little or no scar. Histologically they are typical tuberculous foci and lie in the choriocapillaris. There they can cause alterations in the retinal pigment epithelium and local retinal oedema.

Another form of ocular tuberculosis is the solitary large tubercle of the choroid. This is a very rare occurrence.

119

37—Acquired Syphilitic Choroidoretinitis

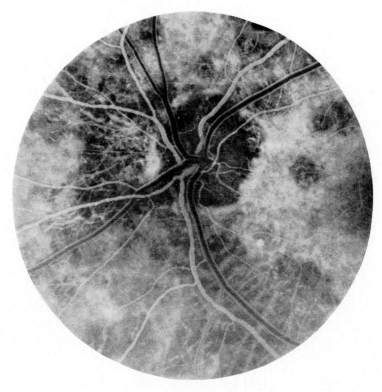

Figure 37

Clinical presentation: White man aged 61 years.

Systemic features: The patient was generally asymptomatic. The ocular findings were suggestive of this disease and the resultant investigation revealed positive serological tests. He successfully underwent a course of treatment with procaine penicillin injections.

Ocular symptoms: The patient had a ten-year history of deterioration of vision. He had been recurrently treated for exacerbations of activity of his choroidoretinitis.

Ophthalmoscopic findings: The left fundus is illustrated in *Plate 37.* The main features are optic atrophy, attenuation of the retinal arteries and widespread pigmentary dispersion.

Fluorescein angiogram: The patchy filling of the choroid with fluorescein (*Figure 37*) is indicative of the areas of atrophy of the choroidal capillaries in particular. The view of this capillary zone is variable as there is dispersion of pigment from the pigment epithelium. Complete areas of non-fluorescence indicate full-thickness choroidal and retinal atrophy. The irregular calibre of all the branches of the central retinal artery would seem to indicate that this patient has also suffered vascular complications of his syphilitic infection.

Finally, the non-fluorescent optic disc shows that its blood supply is markedly diminished as suggested by the ophthalmoscopic findings of optic atrophy.

Additional notes: Congenital choroiditis is one of the leading ocular manifestations of this disease. The appearance of the fundus is very typical and called 'pepper and salt' fundus, because of the fine white and black granules in the fundus. Occasionally this takes the form of bone corpuscle pigmentation.

In acquired syphilis ocular changes only appear in the late stages. The main features are pigmentation in irregular areas together with white atrophic and pigmented scars. Pigment is clumped around veins, especially around branching of veins resulting in 'trousers'.

During periods of active inflammation the retina and choroid have a fluffy whitish appearance and the vitreous is generally cloudy (*see Figure 38*) (with inflammatory cells) over the fundal lesion.

The optic disc may be involved with mild papilloedema and congestive changes.

38—Toxoplasmic Choroidoretinitis

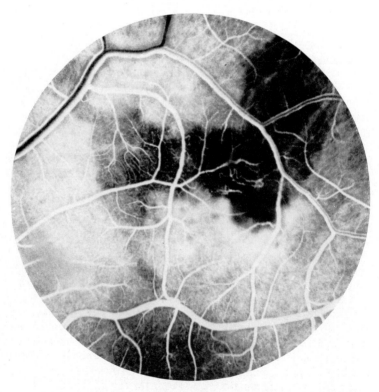

Figure 38 (a)

Clinical presentation: White woman aged 23 years.

Systemic features: None.

Ocular symptoms: Recurrent episodes of blurred vision in the left eye for the past 5 years. Recent onset of a further episode of blurred vision.

Ophthalmoscopic findings: The area of interest was temporal to the optic disc and above the macula and is illustrated in *Plate 38.* A central zone of pigmentary clumping is surrounded by a whitened and fluffy appearance of the retina. This is further surrounded by diffuse retinal oedema with normal fundus seen at the edges of this illustration.

Fluorescein angiogram: Early venous phase (*Figure 38a*) shows the features of a local inflammation in the choroid and retina. The central non-fluorescent area represents the base of the inflammatory process where the pressure from oedema is preventing choroidal perfusion at this site. The lower aspect of the non-fluorescent zone is due to pigmentary clumping. The retinal vessels in the region of the inflammation are generally dilated and leakage of fluorescein is seen particularly adjacent to the non-fluorescent zones. A tributary of the superior temporal vein crossing the zone of inflammation shows calibre variation and irregularity and there are arteriolar and capillary dilatations at the centre of the inflammation. The second angiogram (*Figure 39b*) shows the late-phase appearances when there is persistent fluorescence of the inflammatory exudate. This is the result of retinal vessel leakage of dye in the earlier phases, a consequence of increased permeability in the inflammatory process.

The response of an inflammation of the choroid and retina to treatment can be monitored by fluorescein angiography as it is a most sensitive method of detecting inflammatory activity.

Additional notes: Toxoplasmosis occurs in congenital and acquired forms. In the congenital form, infection occurring early in pregnancy may result in foetal death. Later infection in pregnancy may result in foetal hydrocephalus or microcephalus. Choroidoretinitis occurs in almost 100 per cent of cases of congenital toxoplasmosis. Intracranial lesions acquire later calcification and may readily be identified by radiography.

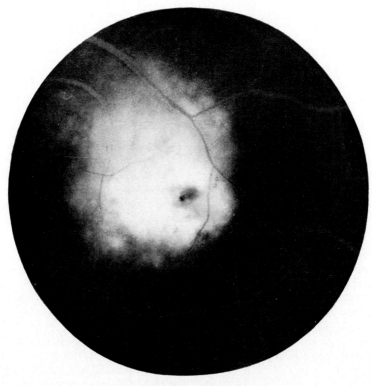

Figure 38 (b)

In the acquired form of toxoplasmosis, choroidoretinal lesions are very rarely accompanied by systemic features. These include exanthematous, lympho-adenopathic and meningitic forms.

39—*Pseudoxanthoma Elasticum*

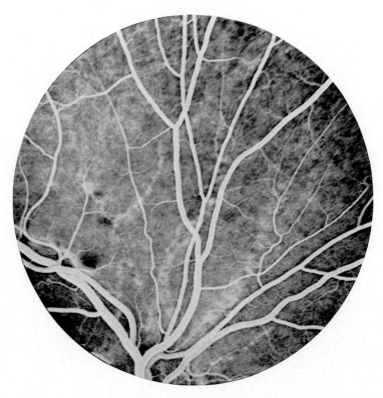

Figure 39

Clinical presentation: White woman aged 23 years.

Systemic features: None.

Ocular symptoms: The patient was asymptomatic but the ocular features, confined to the fundi, were discovered on routine examination.

Ophthalmoscopic findings: The right fundus with the optic disc in the lower portion of the picture is illustrated in *Plate 39,* and the significant features are to be seen in the background of the photograph. In the foreground, retinal arteries and veins radiate from the optic disc. In the background, reddish-brown streaks, roughly following the retinal vessel pattern can be seen. These streaks have a wispy and tortuous configuration. They are known as angioid streaks.

Fluorescein angiogram: Retinal venous phase. The retinal arteries and veins are all brilliantly fluorescent and are easily identified radiating from the region of the optic disc in the lower portion of the picture (*Figure 39*). In the background, the angioid streaks can be identified as hyperfluorescent linear zones which partially merge with the background fluorescence.

These streaks represent cracks or faults in Bruch's membrane, the result of elastic tissue disease. The disruption of Bruch's membrane at these sites is usually associated with a fault in the overlying retinal pigment epithelium. In the long term these faults in Bruch's membrane are replaced by fibrovascular tissue from the choroid.

The angioid streaks become fluorescent coincidentally with appearance of choroidal fluorescence, for this fluorescence is transmitted through the fault in Bruch's membrane and overlying retinal pigment epithelium. According to the state of evolution of the angioid streak, early fluorescence as seen here, may be persistent if there is replacement fibrovascular tissue which tends to stain with fluorescein. In later phase, they will be less fluorescent if they merely transmit late-phase scleral fluorescence.

40—*Pseudoxanthoma Elasticum*

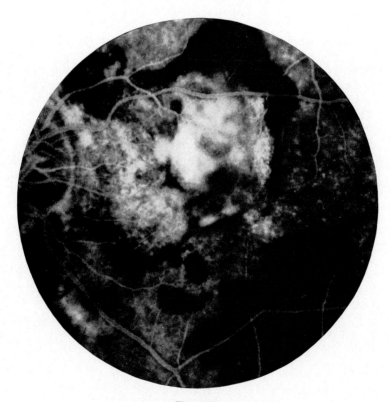

Figure 40

Clinical features: White man aged 38 years.

Systemic features: Recent haematemesis and melaena. Skin changes in neck, axilla and cubital fossae.

Ocular features: Visual acuity 6/5 in the right eye, 6/60 in the left eye. The deterioration in vision in his left eye has been recent—2 months.

Ophthalmoscopic features: Both fundi showed radiating angioid streaks in the region of the optic discs. Additionally, the left fundus showed a macular disturbance. This appeared initially as a greyish elevated area surrounded by a small irregular lake of subretinal haemorrhage. Over a course of several weeks, this appearance changed. The subretinal haemorrhage leaked away or was absorbed, and the central greyish area became more prominent. Thereafter, there was fresh subretinal haemorrhage and yellowish exudates remained where some of this haemorrhage had been absorbed. The left fundus, illustrated in *Plate 40*, is seen some 12 months after onset of visual disturbance. The yellowish grey-green central elevated area is surrounded by scattered hard exudates and subretinal haemorrhage.

Fluorescein angiogram: The subretinal haemorrhage is seen as non-fluorescent areas obscuring choroidal fluorescence but lying beneath the retinal vessels (*Figure 40*). The central raised area is brightly but unevenly fluorescent and elsewhere there is mottled fluorescence in this view.

The mottled fluorescence represents scattered faults in the pigment epithelium, the feature which is sometimes described as an orange-skin (peau d'orange) appearance. The central fluorescent area consists of inflammatory exudate and scar tissue, the result of a central rupture of Bruch's membrane with haemorrhagic and inflammatory consequences. This in turn is the result of elastic tissue degeneration in the lamina of Bruch and represents the macular involvement of the faults, called angioid streaks, seen elsewhere in the fundus.

Additional features: The skin changes, typically on the side of the neck in the axilla and on the forearms, represent elastic tissue degeneration which resembles fatty tissue in appearance, hence the name of the disease as pseudoxanthoma. The elastic tissue degeneration is widespread throughout the body and in particular affects the elastic tissue in blood vessels. Gastro-intestinal haemorrhage may be a serious complication.

41—*Heredopathia Atactica Polyneuritiformis (Refsum's Syndrome)*

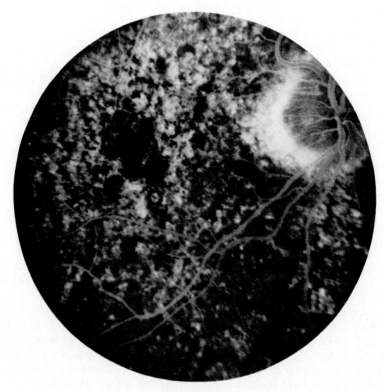

Figure 41

Clinical presentation: White boy aged 16 years.

Systemic features: Progressive polyneuritis with pain and numbness in the hands and feet, followed by muscular weakness and muscle wasting. The patient also suffered from ataxia.

Ocular features: Night blindness and low visual acuity 6/36 in each eye; additionally there was bilateral ptosis.

Ophthalmoscopic findings: Both fundi showed signs of an atypical retinitis pigmentosa. There was a degree of optic atrophy and marked attenuation of all the retinal vessels. Peripheral retinal bone corpuscle pigmentation was prominent; additionally there were signs of macular degeneration. The region illustrated in *Plate 41*, below the right optic disc, shows the general lack of pigment. Choroidal vessels can be seen and a whitish reflection from the sclera is also evident.

Fluorescein angiogram: The same area but also including the macula, is shown in *Figure 41*. This later phase photograph shows the general dispersion of pigment with a resultant mottled fluorescent appearance. This is mainly contributed by scleral fluorescence, which silhouettes surviving pigment cells, choroid and retinal tissue, against it. The irregularity seems to be maximal in the macular region, the principal cause of the patient's low visual acuity.

Additional notes: Onset of night blindness heralds the appearance of an atypical retinitis pigmentosa. Other features of this syndrome include deafness, a polyneuropathy and ataxia. CSF protein levels are usually raised.

The syndrome, which may have a metabolic origin, is inherited as a recessive trait.

42—Laurence-Moon-Bardet-Biedl Syndrome

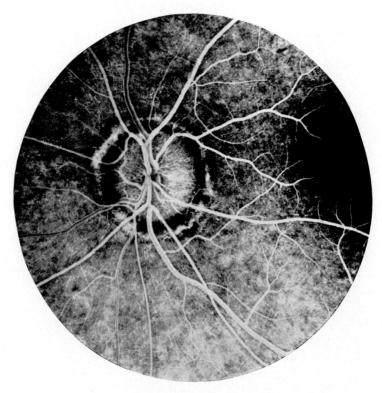

Figure 42

Clinical presentation: White boy aged 14 years.

Systemic features: Patient had 6 fingers on his left hand. There was obesity, mental retardation and cryptorchysm. His sister has polydacly on the left hand.

Ocular features: Ten-year history of deteriorating vision; the initial symptom of defective vision in the dark was followed by defective daylight vision. Acuity was 6/36 in each eye. Visual field testing showed an annular scotoma with a surviving tubular central field of vision and an annular field of peripheral vision.

Ophthalmoscopic findings: The characteristic bone corpuscle pigment aggregates occupied all quadrants of the peripheral retina. These were grouped around retinal blood vessels. The optic disc region, illustrated in *Plate 42*, shows pallor of the disc and some attenuation of the retinal vessels. The greyish appearance of the surrounding fundus is due to pigmentary dispersion.

Fluorescein angiogram: Attenuation of the retinal vessels is shown in the arteriovenous phase angiogram (*Figure 42*). The generalized pigmentary dispersion reveals brilliant fluorescence from the choroid but pigmentary deposits around the optic disc present a non-fluorescent contrast. The radial retinal capillaries are clearly depicted in all quadrants and their continuity with the radiating capillaries on the surface of the optic disc is apparent. Although the disc is clinically pale, the angiogram reveals surprising vascularity although over-emphasis of their quantity is the result of dye leakage from these capillaries giving them undue prominence.

Additional notes: This is a hereditary disease, transmitted as on autosomal recessive, but the genotype is not yet known.

Five leading symptoms belong to this syndrome. (1) Tapetoretinal degeneration, mostly of the retinitis pigmentosa type; (2) polydactyly or syndactyly; (3) mental retardation; (4) obesity; (5) hypogenitalism.

Sometimes other malformations can be found, for example, congenital heart disease, deafness and renal malformations.

The ophthalmoscopic changes are seen only after the age of 4 years. These are bone-corpuscle pigmentation scattered in the mid-periphery of the fundus, arteries which are constricted and the disc which develops a wax-yellow colour.

The night blindness and visual field changes precede fundus changes. The ERG is typically reduced or even extinguished.

133

43—Chloroquine Retinopathy

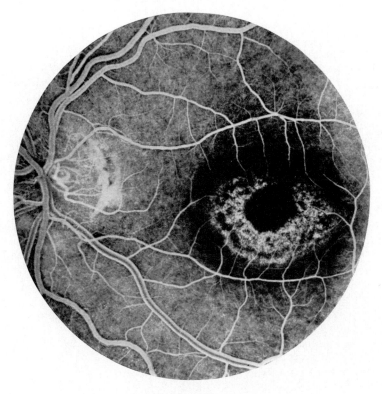

Figure 43

Clinical presentation: White woman aged 59 years.

Systemic features: The patient suffers from chronic rheumatoid arthritis and has been treated with the drug chloroquine for the past 10 years.

Ocular features: The patient had noted deterioration of vision in the left eye more than the right, over the past year. Her acuity was, right eye 6/60, left eye 6/36. Visual field testing revealed a fairly dense central scotoma in each eye.

Ophthalmoscopic findings: The left macular region is illustrated (*Plate 43*). This is the characteristic 'bulls-eye retinopathy' the result of chloroquine therapy over a long term. Migration and aggregation of pigment around the central area contribute to the appearances.

Fluorescein angiogram: Early phase. Fluorescence in the choroid is maximal at this phase, thus faults in the retinal pigment epithelium are highlighted by the underlying fluorescence (*Figure 43*). Pigmentary aggregates block the view of the choroidal fluorescence, whereas pigment dispersion provides a window through a normally densely pigmented layer, to the choroid. The toxic destruction of the retinal pigment epithelium in these central areas is accompanied by destruction of the neurosensory elements at these sites.

Additional notes: This retinopathy occurs in patients under long-term therapy with chloroquine. Only if the dosage is 250 mg or more daily over a period of at least several months do these changes appear, and then only in 1–20 per cent of treated patients.

The first sign is a very fine pigmentary change in the macula which is sometimes reversible. These changes appear in both eyes, but not simultaneously. After some months a depigmented area appears in the macula surrounded by a ring of fine pigmentary granules, giving the impression of a 'bulls-eye'. With time, the retinal vessels show constrictions, bone-corpuscle-like pigmentation appears in the periphery and optic atrophy develops.

The visual field first shows a paracentral scotoma for red, leading to a dense central scotoma. Changes in the ERG or EOG occur prior to the ophthalmoscopic visible changes. Once changes have occurred, recovery is unlikely and cessation of medication may not arrest progression of visual loss.

44—Malignant Melanoma of the Choroid

Clinical presentation: White woman aged 38 years.
Systemic symptoms: None.
Ocular symptoms: Three month history of deteriorating vision in the right eye. Visual acuity 6/60.

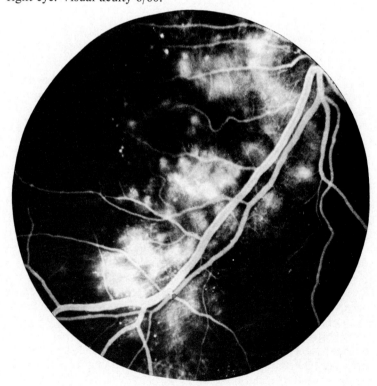

Figure 44

Ophthalmoscopic features: A dark mass irregularly raised from the fundus was found at the temporal side of the optic disc and below (*Plate 44*). Increased pigmentation of the fundus was visible around the disc, and especially towards the macula. No haemorrhage or exudates were seen.

Fluorescein angiogram: Arteriovenous phase. The view, *Figure 44*, is of the inferior temporal retinal vessels with the optic disc above and to the right. Patchy fluorescence around the major vessels and the optic disc contrast with a non-fluorescent background. In the earlier photographs of the angiographic sequence, many dilated capillaries were seen in this field, together with microaneurysms in the retinal circulation. These abnormal vessels were permeable to fluorescein resulting in the staining seen here. Later phase angiograms showed widespread diffusion of the dye and staining of retinal exudates and oedema.

This fundus contained a benign melanoma of the choroid which was very extensive, completely surrounding the optic disc and spreading well beyond the macular region. One portion of this benign melanoma, that is, the inferotemporal zone, had undergone malignant change. The tumour had perforated Bruch's membrane and was causing local embarrassment to the retinal circulation, accounting for the features depicted in the angiogram.

Additional notes: This eye was enucleated and the pathological examination revealed a low-grade malignant melanoma arising from the inferotemporal aspect of a benign melanoma which encircled the optic disc. In the region of malignant change, the overlying choriocapillaries had been largely obliterated and Bruch's membrane was destroyed with malignant tissue invading and replacing the pigment epithelium of the retina. There was shallow detachment of the overlying retina and accumulation of serous exudate in the subretinal space. The retina itself was oedematous and many of the small vessels were dilated. These histological findings confirmed the clinical angiographic interpretation of the exact nature of this disorder.

Malignant melanoma of the choroid is a rare disease but it is the most common of the malignant eye tumours.

The tumour growth starts from the outer layers of the choroid breaking through the Bruch's membrane. The amount of pigment in the tumour is variable. Sometimes a serous retinal detachment, mostly in the lower part of the fundus, is found. Extraocular expansion of these tumours through the sclera is rare. Metastases in the subretinal fluid may cause secondaries in the eye itself, but this is very rare. General metastases especially in the liver are the cause of fatal termination.

137

45—Breast carcinoma metastases in the choroid

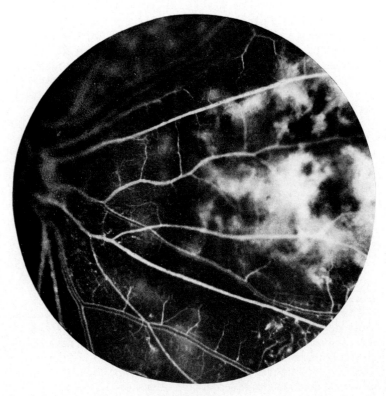

Figure 45

Clinical presentation: White woman aged 49 years.

Systemic features: Six-week history of weight loss, anorexia and loss of energy. The patient had had a radical mastectomy 4 years previously. Clinical examination revealed metastatic deposits in liver and radiographic examination revealed metastatic deposits in the chest. The patient died 3 months later.

Ocular symptoms: Three-month history of deteriorating vision in the right eye.

Ophthalmoscopic findings: On the nasal side of the optic disc, a pale irregularly pigmented elevated plaque-like lesion extended towards the retinal fundus periphery. The area of this region illustrated in *Plate 45*, shows its irregular mottled pallor. Its degree of swelling can be adjudged by the path of the retinal vessels coursing over its surface.

Fluorescein angiogram: Early venous phase. The elevation of this region in the fundus is well shown in the angiogram (*Figure 45*) with its surface in focus and the optic disc to the left of the picture well out of focus in the background. Retinal capillary dilatation and micro-aneurysm formation is occurring as a result of pressure from the tumour beneath. Patchy fluorescence and pigmentation within part of the tumour is well shown.

In the angiographic sequence, this tumour was non-fluorescent in the earliest phase, but having taken up the dye it maintained a mottled fluorescence for several hours.

Additional notes: Metastatic carcinoma of the choroid is the most common of ophthalmic metastases.

The origins are usually breast or bronchus and rarely other sites.

The ophthalmoscopic picture shows an ill-defined raised retinal area over a thickened choroid. Their colour is rather pale grey with a mottled surface. They are localized near the posterior pole, and a serous retinal detachment may appear in association.

The prognosis is naturally poor since it is a sign of dissemination of the primary tumour, but attempts to local treatment are sometimes worth while (irradiation, diathermy or photocoagulation).

46—Von Hippel–Lindau Disease

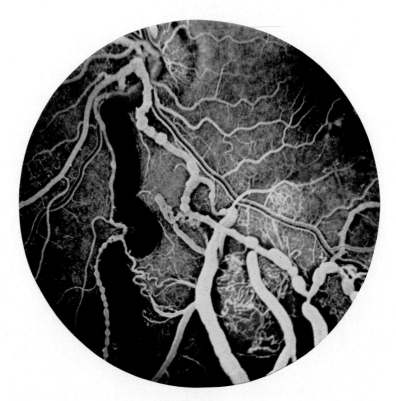

Figure 46

Clinical presentation: White man aged 32 years.

Systemic features: None.

Ocular features: Six-month history of deteriorating vision in the left eye. Visual acuity 6/60.

Ophthalmoscopic findings: Two views, in colour, of the left fundus are illustrated. The first, *Plate 46a,* is of an area well below the optic disc and shows a cherry-like tumour composed of blood vessels. The adjacent retina is detached as can be seen by its colour. An enormously dilated vessel which is very tortuous can be seen on the medial side of the tumour.

The optic disc is just off the upper aspect of the second view (*Plate 46b*), and the tumour seen in the first illustration is just off the lower aspect of this picture, which shows the vascular attachment of the haemangioma. The arterial vessels are grossly distorted having a bead-like appearance. The main artery has enormous fusiform dilatations along its length all the way from the optic disc to the tumour. The main draining vein from the haemangioma is enormously dilated and tortuous, reflecting the high blood flow with which it has to deal. The other feature of this fundus is the retinal exudation; scattered hard exudates are seen throughout the field.

Fluorescein angiogram: The optic disc can be seen at the upper aspect of the picture (*Figure 46*) and emanating from it and descending are the inferior branches of the central retinal artery. The inferotemporal branch of the inferonasal artery descend to supply the haemangioma. The aneurysmal dilatations of these arteries do not require further description. These dilatations are the result of a high intra-arterial blood pressure and flow which in turn is transmitted to the capillary bed deriving from these arteries. As a result, these capillaries are themselves generally dilated and also manifest microaneurysmal dilatations. In the later phase photographs, not illustrated, there is wide-spread leakage of fluorescein from these vessels and staining of this region of the retina. This is reflected in the ophthalmoscopic appearance of the widespread exudation.

It should be noted in *Figure 46* that there is venous return of fluorescein in the inferotemporal retinal vein and the inferonasal retinal vein, whereas the enormously dilated vein which is draining the haemangioma has not yet received any dye which at this time is pooling in the tumour.

141

Additional notes: Von Hippel in 1904 and 1911 described the clinical and pathological features of retinal angiomatosis, a condition with diverse manifestations. In 1926 Lindau noted the frequent occurrence of von Hippel's disease in association with haemangiomas of the cerebellum, kidney, liver and other organs. The combination is, therefore, known as von Hippel–Lindau angiomatosis. Bilateral manifestations in the eyes are said to be present in 50 per cent of cases.

The ocular angiomas undergo progressive changes. The angioma which is probably present at birth often remans dormant until the third or fourth decade of life. It then evolves through enlargement of the angiomatous formation to a stage of haemorrhage and exudation, followed by massive exudation and retinal detachment with ultimate destruction of the eye.

Treatment is possible of the smaller tumours and is best effected by photocoagulation.

Optic Disc Elevation

The causes of optic disc elevation and swelling of the optic nerve head observed by ophthalmoscopic examination include the following.

(1) Raised intracranial pressure.
(2) Raised intra-orbital pressure.
(3) Raised blood pressure.
(4) Retinal vein congestive disorders:
    (a) central retinal vein thrombosis; (b) hyperviscosity syndromes; (c) cardiopulmonary insufficiency.
(5) Papillopathy (Inflammatory Papillitis):
    (a) infective; (b) ischaemic; (c) demyelination; (d) other.
(6) Bone compression of optic nerve:
    (a) traumatic; (b) Paget's disease.
(7) Tumours of optic nerve:
    (a) glioma; (b) meningioma; (c) drusen.
(8) Optic nerve involvement by choroidal tumours:
    (a) haemangioma; (b) melanocytoma; (c) melanoma; (d) metastatic tumour.
(9) Vascular malformations:
    (a) racemose angioma; (b) haemangioma of retina; (c) anomalous arteriovenous communications; (d) anomalous early branching out of retinal vessels.
(10) Anomalous glial proliferation.
(11) Embryonic vascular remnants.
(12) Juxtapapillary subretinal fluid (retinal detachment).

Some of these disorders are of the utmost systemic significance, whereas others have a purely local significance. Although bilateral signs are to be expected in some situations, their asymmetric appearance can cause diagnostic confusion and, similarly, bilateral coincidence of anomalies or absence of one eye may lead to a mistaken diagnosis. Obviously, all symptoms and physical signs are taken into account before a tentative diagnosis is reached. The following notes indicate some helpful ophthalmoscopic and diagnostic features.

The use of stereoscopic colour photography and fluorescein angiography can be extraordinarily helpful in the elucidation of the cause of disc swellings. The precise detail of disc anatomy attained from the magnified, three-dimensional photograph, allied to the additional dynamic information yielded by fluorescein angiography, aids accurate clinical diagnosis.

The retinal photographic service at the United Manchester Hospitals has encouraged referral of cases of diagnostic difficulty with regard to the optic nerve head.

In a two-year period, 1968 and 1969, 77 cases were referred for a photographic assessment of unusual disc elevation. The diagnosis made as a result of this assessment was later borne out by the clinical course of events. The list that follows gives some idea of the clinical problem encountered but it is in no way statistically significant.

Buried drusen in the optic nerve head	15 cases
Anomalous proliferation of glial tissue	4 cases
Vascular malformations	9 cases
Hypermetropia	1 case
Raised intracranial pressure	11 cases
Raised intraorbital pressure	2 cases
Hypertension (malignant)	5 cases
Central retinal vein thrombosis	5 cases
Juxtapapillary choroiditis	6 cases
Acute retrobulbar neuritis	8 cases
Ischaemic optic neuropathy	9 cases
Disc tumour	1 case
Choroid melanoma	1 case
Sarcoidosis	1 case
Still's disease	1 case

(1) *Raised intracranial pressure* is transmitted to the optic nerve by the cerebrospinal fluid in the optic nerve meningeal sheath. When the rise of intracranial pressure is acute, the symptoms and signs are overwhelming and these include papilloedema. From the clinical diagnostic viewpoint it is a slow rise in intracranial pressure and a chronically raised pressure that establishes papilloedema as an such important physical sign. Visual function is only affected in chronic

papilloedema when it has persisted for a period of weeks or months, as a general rule. This is a useful point of differentiation from the 'inflammatory' causes of disc swelling where loss of visual function is a marked and early feature.

Diagnostic features of papilloedema include: elevation of the optic disc, blurring of the disc margins, physiological cupping is often preserved, elevation of tissues beyond the disc margin, dilatation and congestion of vessels on the nerve head; fleck exudates around the swollen disc, haemorrhages on and around the disc. The vessel congestion signs are the earliest changes to appear.

(2) *Raised intraorbital pressure* can cause compression of the orbital venous system with embarrassment of intraocular venous flow. The resultant venous engorgement results in disc oedema and disc swelling. Depending on the severity of the causal condition, some or all of the features of papilloedema in group 1 may appear.

(3) *Raised blood pressure.* Malignant hypertension causes widespread vascular changes in the fundus, including the optic nerve head. Arteriolar necrosis and vessel wall damage from the high intravascular pressure often give rise to gross leakage of plasma and red cells, that is, oedema, exudate and haemorrhage. These changes may be most pronounced at the optic disc region, the most proximal part of the retinal circulation. Retinal oedema merging with disc oedema causes obscuration of the disc margins. Raised intracranial pressure may be a coincidental effect of the hypertension giving a dual mechanism for the papilloedema.

(4) *Retinal vein congestive disorders*

(a) Central retinal vein 'thrombosis' may appear as an isolated phenomenon in an otherwise fit person but more often is associated with arteriosclerotic changes in the central retinal artery. The earliest signs (an incipient thrombosis) of generalized retinal vein congestion proceeds to an overloading situation with haemorrhagic consequences. The full-blown picture is very characteristic, with widespread perivenous dense haemorrhages. Diagnostic confusion usually arises at the earliest stages of this disorder.

(b) Hyperviscosity syndromes, for example, macroglobulinaemia and polycythaemia, are disorders in which circulatory slowing and stasis result in venous and capillary congestion with haemorrhage, oedema and lipid deposits. Bilateral signs make confusion with the papilloedema of raised intracranial pressure a possibility. Haematological investigation, which reveals the diagnosis, must always be considered in relation to the clinical findings of disc swelling.

145

(c) Cardiopulmonary insufficiency occurring in patients with emphysema, cor pulmonale and poor ventilation in extreme obesity, all have carbon dioxide retention. Papilloedema is a common finding in this situation.

(5) *'Inflammatory' causes of disc swelling (Papillitis)*

(a) *Infective.*—Choroiditis adjacent to the optic disc—juxtapapillary choroiditis—is sometimes difficult to diagnose in the early stages. An early sign is disc swelling which may be apparent before a juxtapapillary focus of inflammatory activity becomes obvious. Equally, the overflow into the vitreous of inflammatory cells and exudate may not occur immediately to help identify the nature of the lesion. The infecting agent may be hard to define but toxoplasmosis is the most common. Disc swelling as a component of generalized fundus oedema does not often give rise to diagnostic difficulties regarding differentiation from papilloedema. However, disc swelling as a feature of a posterior uveitis is found in Behçet's disease, Harada's disease and sarcoidosis. There remains a possibility that these disorders have an infective origin. Tuberculous and syphilitic choroidoretinitis belong to this group of infective causes of disc swelling.

(b) *Ischaemic.*—Atherosclerosis, embolism or arteritis may result in arteriolar occlusion in relation to the blood supply of the optic nerve head. Deriving its main arterial supply from the adjacent choroid, occlusive disease of the short posterior ciliary arteries or their feeding arterioles to the optic nerve head gives rise to the clinical condition of ischaemic optic neuropathy. Systemic associations can include diabetes mellitus and herpes zoster ophthalmicus.

(c) *Demyelination.*—Acute retrobulbar neuritis is an early manifestation of multiple sclerosis. It is usually transient and its effects reversible. About 40 per cent of all cases of multiple sclerosis contract a retrobulbar neuritis at some stage. Up to 40 per cent of all young adults who present with an acute retrobulbar neuritis, in due course develop other symptoms and signs of multiple sclerosis.

The ophthalmoscopic picture varies from normal disc and fundus appearances, approximately 50 per cent, to a gross papilloedema with some retinal oedema. Those fundi which have a normal ophthalmoscopic appearance may have an abnormal fluorescein angiogram (*see Figure 8*), dye leakage and tissue staining identifying a 'sub-clinical' papilloedema. Acute retrobulbar neuritis has a typical clinical picture which includes pain on eye movement, globe tenderness and a central scotoma in the field of vision which may extend to give a temporary state of no light perception.

(d) *Other causes* include 'toxic papilloedema, for example, due to tetracycline.

(6) *Bone compression of the optic nerve*

Trauma.—Disc oedema and haemorrhage can result from compression of the optic nerve in the optic canal as it passes from the orbit into the cranium, if the optic canal is fractured in a head injury. Unless relief of the compression is carried out rapidly, irreversible optic atrophy will ensue.

Paget's disease.—The bony compression of the optic nerve passing through the optic canal is a gradual process in Paget's disease. Disc changes may therefore present as a clearly progressive optic atrophy or alternatively as papilloedema. In the latter case it is difficult to decide whether this phenomena is purely the result of nerve compression or of concurrently raised intracranial pressure, also the result of bone changes in the skull. Bilateral signs may be helpful as well as other neurologic symptoms, signs and radiographic findings. Osteopetrosis, Albers–Schönberg disease can produce optic atrophy following oedema of the disc due to optic nerve compression in the optic canal.

(7) *Tumours of the optic nerve*

Glioma.—This tumour may present with congestive signs in the optic disc and retina, that is, papilloedema with associated proptosis of the globe. The more insidious course of events results in slowly progressive optic atrophy.

Angioma of the optic nerve sheath.—These occur even more rarely than gliomas, and are more difficult to treat. Their symptomatology is very similar to the glioma with papilloedema giving rise to subsequent optic atrophy.

Drusen.—Hyaline or colloid bodies in the fundi. The term drusen is derived from the Czechoslovak 'druza' meaning a cavity in a cliff filled with crystals. These bodies may be small, large, multiple, buried or superficial in relation to the optic nerve head.

A clinical diagnosis of buried drusen in the optic nerve head is supported by: (1) an irregular swelling of the optic disc; (2) an irregular disc margin; (3) an amorphous appearance of the disc elevation; (4) drusen elsewhere in the same fundus, the other eye, or optic discs of close relatives.

Buried drusen in the optic nerve head of children may become visible in adult life. Familial occurrence of drusen is recognized as an irregular dominant hereditary affection.

(8) *Optic nerve head involvement by choroidal tumours*

Haemangiomas.—These tumours, as elsewhere in the body, are present in some form at birth and may suddenly undergo active enlargement in the third, fourth and fifth decades of life. Exudative phenomena are associated with the local haemodynamic alterations which result from the active expansion of the lesion. By ophthalmoscopy, a choroidal haemangioma may appear as a relatively circumscribed swelling with associated retinal and subretinal lipid deposits and oedema. These exudative and congestive changes can involve the optic nerve head inducing disc swelling.

Melanocytoma.—This term is given to the malignant melanoma which grows in the optic nerve head, causing a pigmented swelling of the optic disc. It is believed to originate in the adjacent choroid.

Large tumours.—Large tumours in the choroid, melanomas and metastatic tumours can cause congestive changes in the optic nerve head, by direct pressure.

(9) *Vascular malformations*

Racemose angioma.—The generalized involvement of the retinal blood vessels in the angiomatous process. Tortuosity, looping, excessive branching and engorgement of vessels are typical features. The optic disc may be obscured by such an anomaly, the congestive appearance and exudative phenomena can be suggestive of papilloedema.

Haemangioblastoma.—Capillary haemangiomas forming cherry-like tumours are occasionally located in the optic disc region. Their mis-diagnosis as papilloedema has occurred on numerous occasions. Fluorescein angiographic appearances are diagnostic.

Anomalous early branching of retinal vessels and *anomalous arteriovenous communications* can simulate papilloedema.

(10) *Anomalous glial proliferation.—See* para. 11 below.

(11) *Embryonic vascular remnants.* The occurrence may be unilateral or bilateral. Persistence of the embryonic vascular system of the inner eye, the hyaloid system may be in the form of a cyst, called Bergmeister's papilla or a persistent frond of vessels overlying the optic disc. Associated with these vascular remnants, glial supporting tissue contributes to the disc elevation. Glial proliferation may also occur in the absence of vascular remnants, its cause unknown.

(12) *Juxtapapillary subretinal fluid.* The presence of subretinal fluid, adjacent to the optic disc, in retinal detachment, causes distinct blurring of the disc margin and the elevation of the retinal vessels can result in misdiagnosis of papilloedema. This is a reminder that an ophthalmoscopic examination should not be confined to the region of the optic disc.

Index